Death before Dying

Death before Dying

GARY S. BELKIN

NEW YORK UNIVERSITY SCHOOL OF MEDICINE

NEW YORK, NY

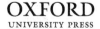

OXFORD

UNIVERSITY PRESS

Oxford University Press is a department of the University of Oxford.
It furthers the University's objective of excellence in research, scholarship,
and education by publishing worldwide.

Oxford   New York
Auckland   Cape Town   Dar es Salaam   Hong Kong   Karachi
Kuala Lumpur   Madrid   Melbourne   Mexico City   Nairobi
New Delhi   Shanghai   Taipei   Toronto

With offices in
Argentina   Austria   Brazil   Chile   Czech Republic   France   Greece
Guatemala   Hungary   Italy   Japan   Poland   Portugal   Singapore
South Korea   Switzerland   Thailand   Turkey   Ukraine   Vietnam

Oxford is a registered trademark of Oxford University Press
in the UK and certain other countries.

Published in the United States of America by
Oxford University Press
198 Madison Avenue, New York, NY 10016

© Oxford University Press 2014

Library of Congress Cataloging-in-Publication Data
Belkin, Gary S. (Gary Stuart), 1962– author.
[Death before dying (Oxford University Press)]
Death before dying / Gary Belkin.
p.; cm.
Includes bibliographical references.
ISBN 978–0–19–989817–6 (alk. paper)
I. Title.
[DNLM: 1. Brain Death.   2. Bioethical Issues.   3. Consciousness. W820]
RA427.25
174.2—dc23
2013033106

9 8 7 6 5 4 3 2 1
Printed in the United States of America
on acid-free paper

To all of those whose lives have been interrupted
by hard medical decisions

CONTENTS

ACKNOWLEDGMENTS

This book would not have happened without a confluence of generous circumstances and generous people who let me translate a personal passion for history into a PhD and subsequent deep dive into this subject. While in training as a resident in psychiatry at Massachusetts General Hospital (MGH) in the early 1990s, I was three subway stops away from the Harvard University Department of the History of Science. MGH (in the form of John Herman) and Harvard (personified in a troika of cherished mentors: Everett Mendelsohn, Barbara Rosenkrantz, and Allan Brandt) made it possible to leverage that proximity along with small patches of flexible time into a workable pathway toward completing the requisite coursework. It was during this time that I started to gather some of the material presented here, revisiting it all well over a decade later at the urging of my wife, Kate, who thought that perhaps some better use could be made of this research than as the basis for random intrusions into dinner conversations. She turned out (as usual) to be right. For her encouragement and for many other, even better reasons, I am grateful for every day that she is in my life.

Thoughtful readings of the whole or parts of versions of the manuscript from Daniel Callahan, Barron Lerner, David Millett, and Eelco Wijdicks were very much appreciated, as was the belief, from Craig Panner at Oxford University Press that this was worth doing, even through my shameless moving of deadlines.

It has been some time since I put them to work, but I am eternally grateful to the staff at the MGH Medical Records Department who repeatedly came through for me and who were remarkably adventurous in tracking down, from remote storage, records from the 1950s and 1960s. I am deeply grateful for the opportunity to have met Robert Schwab's long-time collaborator Mary Brazier, and his widow Joan Schwab, both of whom shared valuable recollections as well as otherwise unobtainable papers of Robert Schwab. The recollections of other formative participants or witnesses to many of the events described here also include Raymond Adams, C. Miller Fisher, Edward Lowenstein, Vincent Perlo, Henning Pontoppidan, Joseph Murray, William Sweet, and Robert Young. Many of their specific comments are dutifully referenced in these pages but their time to share an overall sense of working at MGH during this period was much appreciated for thinking about the themes that formed this book. My gratitude also goes to Jessica Murphy at the Center for the History of Medicine at the Countway Library of Medicine, who was wonderfully flexible in making materials there available, and to Fred Plum for his insights on what we can know about coma. Thanks as well to Keith Chiappa who miraculously uncovered hidden cabinets of old microfilmed EEG recordings at MGH, and Anne Harrington for one of those tipping-point seed grants that got me the person-hours of help I needed to sift through over ten thousand tracings on those microfilms. I was also privileged to train under Ned Cassem, who brought me onto the MGH Optimum Care Committee he created thirty years earlier; this is where I first took on the task of diagnosing brain death and of trying to make sense of difficult end-of-life and other care decisions with patients, families, and caregivers.

The contribution of a few neighborhood cafés, and their passion for making espresso a true craft, should not be underestimated and provided me with invaluable workspace (and attention enhancement) over several years. Thank you Jonathan Rubinstein (Joe!), Sam Penix (Everyman!), and the whole crew at Stumptown. Thanks to Kira—for looking over this earlier on and being honest that it needed a do over; to Lisa—for showing me so skillfully that Belkins can write books; and to Mom and Al—for being proof that lifelong learning is the fountain of youth. Richard Jennis has helped keep me afloat for over three decades now, and Amanda Davidson helped me be clearer and get closer to rules of grammar and prose I otherwise tend to ignore.

Finally, Annie and Emma: I am not sure how much of my own romance with history will rub off on you. But the work of writing history would do well with no higher goal than to help move the world a bit closer toward the integrity and humanity you each already have. You are deeply loved.

INTRODUCTION: FEAR AND TREMBLING

"I have pronounced many individuals dead, and, believe me, I am nervous and on edge when I do."

—EDWIN H. ALBANO, *New Jersey Medical Examiner, September, 1968*

"When all is said and done, it seems ironic that the end point of existence, which ought to be as clear and sharp as in a chemical titration, should so defy the power of words to describe it and the power of men to say with certainty, "It is here.""

—EDITORIAL, *JAMA, 1968*

"More and more, we are going to die when someone makes the decision that we are going to die."

—*The New York Times, February 2, 1997*

My first night as a doctor began with a request to declare a patient dead. Unexpectedly, a question came to mind: How do I *know* this person is dead? On the one hand, I was fairly confident that his heart was no longer beating, that he was no longer breathing, and that he was, dead. But when handed the task of formal declaration—of officially and permanently drawing the line he had crossed—I hesitated. Initially, that hesitation centered on deciding which method would best verify this apparent absence of pulse and breathing. I sought evidence of the slightest movement of heart and lungs as the magnitude of my pronouncement sunk in. How was I *sure*? Should I get an electrocardiogram (ECG)? In fact, I did get an ECG, and obsessed some more over the accuracy of my examination. But as the initial uncertainty receded, another took its place. I was confident in my physical findings, but how did they translate into a notion of death? What did that label *mean*, and did my findings clearly add up to such a meaning?

Since then, an additional consideration came to mind: Was the question of meaning, however fascinating, relevant to the task at hand? That final question loomed larger as I later became a more focused student of history and looked at debates over the appearance of an alternative definition of death that emerged in the late 1960s—brain death—through that lens. A strange combination of certainty and lingering pause, of natural "fact" and metaphysical speculation, has always swirled around the task of defining death. Not surprisingly, a vast body of literature is devoted to examining brain death's meanings and conceptual features. But whether these kinds of questions about medicine's "meanings" get us closer to addressing the challenges of connecting medical practice with our values seemed to me to be less clear.

"Brain death" is a fascinating medical fact. For one thing, it remains controversial and debated despite also being widely and routinely used as criteria for declaring death around the world. What do we make of the scenario where something presumably so clear—the time of death—should remain controversial and uncertain half a century after the Ad Hoc Committee of the Harvard Medical School to Examine the Definition of Brain Death and its chairman, Massachusetts General Hospital (MGH) anesthesiologist Henry K. Beecher, proposed to define it in a Report published in 1968?[1] Criticism of brain death criteria began with criticism of the Committee's work. This book revisits the sources for the Harvard Committee's Report and essentially makes two arguments. The first is to challenge prevailing historical characterizations of the Report as ethically unsophisticated, problematically focused on transplantation, and lacking a conceptual justification and empirical basis for this way of understanding and defining death. The second is to describe why correcting this history is important. It is important, briefly, because these prevailing characterizations have tended to rest on drawing a distinction between medical knowledge, and ethical expertise over its use; between medical facts themselves, and the values implicit in them. If the history needs revision, perhaps these driving assumptions about how to relate ethics to medicine do as well. Challenging each historical characterization allows room for a different focus—a focus on alternatives to a distinct ethics-perspective for managing the value dimensions and consequences of medical facts. Taking on some of the roots of controversy over the fact of brain death opens up larger questions about how to approach the value dimensions of medical facts, and of healthcare more generally.[2]

Since the Report appeared in the United States, the criteria were reviewed and endorsed by presidential commissions in 1981 and again in 2008, and were updated and adopted by the American Neurological Association in 1995 and 2010.[3] Yet the past half-century has also seen continual challenges to the credibility and appropriate justification of these criteria. Brain death was an early target of a group of American intellectuals in the late 1960s and early 1970s who claimed that since medicine was a source of ethics and values, it needed to be managed with the study and application of ethics expertise. A growing network of analysis, literature, review processes, and oversight mushroomed from this claim over the following decades under the umbrella of "bioethics." Eventually, institutionalized responsibilities for ethics review and oversight were implemented within healthcare institutions ranging from the World Health Organization to every hospital in the United States. No aspect of human experience or culture, other than perhaps formal religious practice, has likely witnessed routinized application of "ethics" of this intensity. Why, and to what effect?

Fascination with tidying up deep and unruly questions of what life essentially means is understandable, but looking over the cumulative result of decades of such debate over brain death proves disappointing. There has been very little change in the basic terms of this debate, which reads as a relentlessly circular conversation, dissecting the conceptual groundings for a definition of brain death. This effort to define the essential concept of what we call "death" was elusive, and not clearly productive.

The Report, and initial efforts that would herald the appearance of bioethics as a field, engaged each other early on. So the unfolding of the brain death debate is a good place to start to ask these questions about ethics and medicine. That medical facts could be contingent and carry values and meanings was not a new insight, and it was voiced frequently by Beecher among others. Joseph Fletcher—a friend and confidante of Beecher's, a theologian and public intellectual who engaged early on the implications of health technologies for moral values, and a strong proponent of using brain death criteria—wrote, soon after the Harvard Report appeared: "The picture of what has happened in the technology of medicine and paramedical care fills us, ambivalently, with fear and confidence, assurance and doubt— both as to the facts themselves and as to the value-meaning of the facts, their ethical significances."[4] Should medical *facts* define important *meanings*? Are these facts and explanations merely data and free of meaning, or do they, and should they, broker choices over core values?

The asserted need to draw distinctions between medical facts and values lay at the heart of early bioethical critiques of brain death, and justified the routine use of expertise about values and ethics to inform and shape how medicine and research are practiced, and how dilemmas in care are resolved. This book suggests that this strategy failed when looked at through the lens of brain death. The ways in which brain death made sense as a medical fact to those who first described it in detail provides an opportunity to consider alternative strategies for managing value-laden, contingent, and iterative medical facts.

How did I *know* that man I was called to see was dead? To answer that I recognize that I could "know" in the sense of mere data, of a fact made plain because of its tangible, interobserver reliable features. I could also know through connections I make in what those features mean or associations and values I put into them. Especially in the medical context, those ways of knowing are inextricably talking to each other. The designation and distinction between the categories of "the normal and the pathological" require that exchange.[5] How biological signs are consigned to normalcy or to pathology is steeped in mere data from the body, but also in how those data turn out to instrumentally work for us to do things. Lived experience and mere data push back on each other in ongoing, iterative fashion, continuously remaking what we can, or want to, reduce to medical data.

Keeping pace with the walking biological creatures that we are requires, if not demands, a pragmatic point of view of medical knowledge, as well as of medical values. Paying attention to how medical knowledge yields predictions and solves problems is a foundational starting point for describing the values surrounding it. Brain waves, physical examination, and other building blocks and signals used to describe the working brain, for example, are integral to the moral valence of describing brain death as death. How these "mere data" were composed and worked with other mere data set limits on the perceived or allowable scope of credible medical action, and of possible descriptions for death and dying. Bending medical facts towards purposes we value requires a deeper curiosity than work in bioethics has tended to bring to bear about how medical knowledge works, and the tools it has to work with.

The explosive growth of bioethics was a response to a loss of faith in the pragmatism of the medical point of view, of the thought style and structure of medical knowledge as a source of values. Paradoxically, the spread of bioethics did little to alter the spread of biomedical power and instead, some have argued, fueled it. At least in the case of brain death, attempts to split off and separate analysis of value from analysis of fact failed to rein in the power of mere biomedical data. Work in bioethics may have started from pointing out the composite fact–value nature of medical facts, but did not take it seriously *enough*. History matters in all this. It has frequently been used to support a story of the necessity of bioethics to solve dilemmas in medicine. That use of history has eclipsed other possibilities for history to be better used to understand how medical knowledge works, and point to more effective ways to improve it.

Moral or ethical claims about how medical providers should act, or what patients deserve, or whether brain death is credible, have traction to the degree they match up, not along ethical categorization or rules of moral philosophical argument, but along the constraints and possibilities of practice and knowledge that come from probing and querying the body. The challenge may be made that in making that point I argue the limits of ethics but use one of its tools to do so—that it sounds like I may be choosing Pragmatism as one ethical or philosophical position over others, and that I need to justify that position. Indeed I will refer, as Beecher himself did, to Beecher's pragmatism. I resist, though, the assumption that making that point is a philosophical claim. We can observe people acting and knowledge working pragmatically. It is possible to make that point as an observation, which is consistent with the findings of this history, not as a philosophical claim. If such an observation turns out to fall within one philosophical subject heading or another, that is an accident. It does not provide a basis for agreement or disagreement.

As it is possible to base conversations about the purposes of medicine by starting with curiosity about the structure of medical knowledge itself without signing up for a particular school of ethical thinking, it is also possible to do so without, at the other extreme, descending into pure naturalism or scientism. This is something both liberal and conservative bioethicists often fear. Avoiding that was something Beecher actually explicitly voiced. It is a justified fear, one that has long complicated political and cultural support of science and scientific stewardship of social and technological progress, but it is one that has arguably been best wrestled with pragmatically, rather than morally.[6] The ability to define what kind of healthcare is "better" "equitable," or "just" will require more attention to how to leverage the pragmatic learning internal to medicine differently, and less attention to either expert-detailed or slogan-inspired moralized categories and language. Our ability to make that shift has large consequences. It may ultimately determine whether the use of medical knowledge in modern societies is affordable, accessible, or effective.

A careful history of brain death proves useful for exploring this larger context. This is especially so because of the degree to which historical characterizations have tended to reinforce what the emerging bioethics discipline wanted to hear about the idea of ethical experts arbitrating the consequences of living in a biomedical culture. Within the field of bioethics, the historical characterizations of bioethics and of brain death have tended to support each other along a shared narrative trajectory. This narrative first describes bioethics as a needed rescue from the ways that medicine masked as objective facts what were really moral choices. Second, brain death was a perfect example of how badly medicine needed bioethics in this way. After all, critics argued, the practices comprising brain death were not only moral choices, beyond the purview of physicians. These practices also appeared to be attempts, on the part of physicians, to hide what should be public agendas, in this case to expand transplantation and access to organs without direct public sanction.

Neither of these aspects of the narrative hold up to scrutiny. This book focuses on the work of key members of the Harvard Committee in the decades preceding their Report and challenges the usual storyline of the Committee as unduly invested in transplantation. Instead, the book explores how brain death architects arguably engaged many of the same issues that the bioethical narrative lays unique claim to. Correcting, or at least complicating the history of brain death therefore complicates a prevailing narrative of bioethics as the go-to strategy for managing complex medical facts, thereby opening new routes of consideration for how to manage biomedical dilemmas.

A revised history of brain death provides an entry point, then, for reimagining the core concerns of bioethics including autonomy, paternalism, beneficence, experiment, progress, and agency in medicine, reframing these as enduring and, in essence, morally ambiguous, practices. Rather than belonging to the discipline of ethics, these core concerns can be understood and treated as the result of historically specific conditions of practice and as features of complex applied medical knowledge.

These broader conclusions emerged from exploring historical questions specific to this book: What were the experiences and purposes of the original architects of the definition of brain death? What was the context of medical practice within which this new definition made sense? Answers came in part from medical records at MGH in the 1950s and 1960s detailing the care of hundreds of patients with coma—the data and experience from which the Harvard definition essentially emerged. Answers also arose from consideration of chairman Henry Beecher's attitudes and actions with respect to rules for human experimentation, especially in the context of 1960s debates over moral theology and the challenges of secularism and social change. These sources described a quite different historical narrative of the Committee, and so led to my own confrontation with the assumptions and history that anchor the bioethical project. In the field of bioethics and in medical humanities scholarship, the prevailing characterization of the Committee's work as medicine-run-amok did not add up. I found Beecher's justification for the Committee to be grounded in considerations of ethics and, more importantly—and instructively—in dilemmas arising from challenges in the use and generation of medical knowledge, especially experimental knowledge. Given these expanded considerations, bioethics in general—and criticisms of brain death in particular—appeared less as a solution than an anachronism, a fetish over moral meanings actually ill-equipped to handle the values, fears, attitudes, and expectations that drive dilemmas in healthcare.

Among those attitudes were strangeness and ambivalence. For some healthcare providers and families, the option of declaring brain death allowed for a humane course of action; while for others, brain death carried the sinking feeling that they were in over their heads. Should anyone dare assert control over the nature of life when it seemed (and continues to seem) so strange to do so? Palpably and repeatedly rehearsed within medicine, these tensions—between extremes of comfort and strangeness, relief and foreboding, knowledge and skepticism, fact and metaphysics, choice and fate, resentment and comfort—have accelerated considerably throughout the twentieth century and continue to gain momentum at the outset of the new millennium, as our capacities for manipulating our genes or our neuronal circuitry seem to only be warming up. Twentieth-century and early twenty-first-century Western societies in particular are, increasingly, biomedical cultures. And yet the unavoidable disconnect between everyday lived experience and, conversely, our experiences as medical subjects or biological objects creates anxiety, wariness, and ambivalence alongside the hope often attached to advancing medical routines and prerogatives.

This enduring and intense ambivalence that drove the flight into ethics deserves more attention. On the one hand, medicine was—and is—faulted for too often offering marginal benefits while risking prolonged suffering with intrusive, intensive, technological capabilities and manipulative powers over the body. On the other hand, these same capabilities continue to be desperately and widely sought as a source of great benefit, comfort, and progress. They are yearned for and also guarded against. Despite the scrutiny of physician authority that began to grow in the mid-1960s, *biomedical* authority—that is, the broader use of biomedical methods, expertise, vocabularies, and sciences to explain who we are and how we are doing—persisted, if not flourished. Biomedicine's stock rose higher as that of physicians' declined through the end of the twentieth century and into the twenty-first.

We manage these complex expectations wth complex facts. The peculiar suspension of nonsentient human life made possible by respirators and other intensive care technology from the 1950s onward lent urgency to the task of describing or defining death as a standard, criteria-based fact. While intense wariness over the strangeness of the comatose body helped fuel ethical scrutiny over medicine, the mix of implicit meanings and pragmatic purposes attributed to the new phenomenon of brain death were (and are) common—if not essential—to other medical facts whose definitions are intended to provide more predictability and actionability in managing our biological selves. These include less dramatic negotiations such as setting appropriate frequency for screening mammography, establishing cutoffs for high cholesterol, or ranking the effectiveness of sequential choices of chemotherapy. These practices may not be as rich in existential meaning as defining death, but they too present the common, if not unavoidable, contingency and value dimensions of medical facts.

Managing the ambiguity of the uniquely "modern fact," one that could be "represented either as mere data…or as data gathered in the light of a social or theoretical context that made them seem worth gathering," is a core task of modern capitalist societies.[7] This task is central to the uses and misuses of public health and investments in healthcare. We need histories and other tools to learn and be curious (and demanding) about this contingency and complexity of medical facts, both as mere data and as instruments for action within specific contexts. At least with respect to the debates over brain death, much of the work attributed to bioethics did not yield new learning or knowledge. It instead tended to confuse cleverness with new knowledge, reflection with action, and analysis with actual solutions. When bioethics did make real impact, such as defining now widely used procedures for review of research and informed consent, it did so through precisely the kinds of technocratic routines it originally set out to reject.[8]

This book arrives at these larger themes starting from a smaller focus— how to make sense of hundreds of medical records that describe the care of comatose patients at MGH in the decade leading up to the Report. That care was very much influenced by a key architect of the specific criteria announced in the Report: Robert Schwab, who was a colleague of Beecher's and a neurologist at MGH. These records, along with the medical and legal literature on coma of the time, capture the cautiousness and complexity of the movement within hospital-based medical practice to adopt and name brain death criteria in response to what I call the experience of "death before dying." This term describes the quite new and distinct ability, emerging through the 1950s and 1960s, to act on bodies in the medical context in a way that suspended functioning, brought an expanded scope of manipulative power to medicine, and markedly separated metabolic and cardiovascular physiology, from the nervous system.

The Report was an early attempt to navigate this new world of death before dying by setting standards that could guide medical care using rules chosen for simplicity, reproducibility, and transparency. This framing places the Committee in the context of developments in the management and scrutiny of healthcare over the following half-century that focused less on meanings and morals than on outcomes, accountability, and the properties of medical evidence. Here, too, is a potential alternative historical perspective on how values in healthcare are connected to—if not dependent upon—the management, definition, and use of medical knowledge in practice. The inadequacies of the bioethical project in the case of brain death underscore the importance and complexity of medical facts as carriers of values, and the need for deeper curiosity about the workings of medical knowledge as a source for values. The bioethical critique may have generally gotten the order and dynamic wrong in terms of how values and knowledge relate. The consequences of this misprioritization are significant in terms of what ethicists, practitioners, and the public ought to really worry about, improve, and debate regarding the purposes of medicine. Practices precede ethics. The latter is incomprehensible without the former. This is not stated as an ideological position but as a feature and consequence of working with the body in a powerful kind of effort to heal it. This history starts there, with practice, and with the historical context of the medical knowledge and workings in which the dilemma of brain death surfaced.

OUTLINE

I approached the Report curious as to how it was put together. How did it make sense to those who wrote it? Chapter One outlines the perspectives and experiences that some physicians, such as Beecher, used to develop and articulate their concerns about increasingly intrusive medical practices. Responses to "hopeless" cases and "heroic" treatment in the decades leading up to the Report built upon longstanding concerns within and without medicine over extraordinariness of care, the nature of experiment, and the demands of truth-telling. Beecher inherited and also reshaped that context as he connected facts about the body with the rights of patients. Together, these issues led him to see the necessity of defining brain death. His justification for doing so is described in more detail in Chapter Two, as are the views of his critics. Beecher's justification is perhaps best explained within the context of his experiences with human experimentation. Ultimately, brain death marked the line that separated acceptable medical care and unacceptable experimentation. For his critics, the salient issues were quite different. But Beecher and his critics were actually joint participants in debates over the scope, uses, and limits of ethics.

Understanding other sections of the Report require revisiting, on the one hand, a long tradition of case law on the timing of death and, on the other, an evolving body of research and related clinical practice with respect to consciousness and coma beginning in the 1920s. Chapter Three focuses on the first issue: the background of case law that was referenced in a section of the Report which addressed the legal standing of the Committee's efforts. That tour of case law reinforces the uniqueness and impact of death before dying and offers evidence of a broader interest among some legal scholars in new solutions—such as brain death—to address it. Chapters Four and Five discuss the medical records of patients with flat or markedly diminished EEG findings who were seen by Schwab and his EEG lab during his tenure at MGH. These chapters also examine the rapid growth in EEG-based research, which offered a new, though uncertain, medical language for understanding human consciousness.

This material addresses often-criticized ambiguities in the Report: the lack of clarity as to whether it was attempting to define a certain kind of coma or death itself and, relatedly, its lack of a clear conception of *life*, the end of which was signaled by brain death. Critics of the Report have seen this lack of explicit conceptual grounding as a (suspicious) weakness. However, in revisiting the background of clinical experience and EEG-based research that shaped Schwab's criteria, such ambiguities can be seen to reflect, instead, a combinatory logic—one that brought together a version of situation ethics that Beecher explicitly endorsed; a consideration of the sorts of patients Schwab and his colleagues faced; the state of knowledge about the neurology of consciousness; and an attempt to reconcile ambiguity through practice standards.

After revisiting the evidence, sources, and experiences that the Report's authors actually drew upon—material rarely if ever explored among the truckloads of commentary on brain death—the book then looks at events since the Report's appearance. Chapter Six picks up some of the more provocative themes I began with here. The book closes by thinking about how these themes might draw us to different solutions for taking on the fact–value juggernaut of medicine, especially given its continued trajectory toward a future of neurological manipulation and in light of the expanding domain of neuroscience and cognitive science in explaining people, society, and culture.

The respirator was arguably a first tangible step in bionic therapeutics, and one that profoundly altered the nature of medicine's manipulative power—a development as far-reaching as other key milestones such as the use of anesthesia. The discomfort and consequences of the emergence of death before dying are still with us. Unnerved by that, ethics critics at the time focused on an apparent divide between alienating medicalization and autonomous conscious choice.

That response may have captured anxiety over medical power but offered limited options for meeting it. Although "neuroethics" appeared in the 1990s to address some of the similar accelerating set of anxieties about brain-based manipulation, it resembles its bioethical namesake too closely, so far, to be other than a distraction—in essence, more of the same. Neuroethics may similarly miss the mark in getting at deeper change to medical practice—particularly in managing costly, technologically intensive, intrusive medicine that can itself be a symptom of a highly consequential ambivalence about embodiment and medical facts that needs to be approached head-on through critical examination of that knowledge, its properties, and sources.

The turn to ethics, the *conceptual turn*, may have instead diminished the possibilities for a more robust medical humanism with which to help do that. Ethics and its application of moral philosophical tools comes too late to the medical dilemmas it looks to solve. Ethical terms describe what these dilemmas look like, but do not critically explore or explain as well as other options in the medical humanities and social sciences toolkit where and how they originated, or can be comprehensively addressed. History—and anthropology, sociology, epidemiology, psychology, political science—engages that more directly.[9]

In this history of brain death, medical practice appears as a more complex and potential source for framing norms and values and providing a foundation for its own transformation than it has been given credit for, or that we have learned to effectively use. Medical knowledge describes, predicts, and manipulates biological mechanisms. This inevitably creates tension with the other sources of knowledge and meaning that we use to understand and live our lives. This book, though, questions whether drawing on a distinct form of ethical reasoning or moral philosophy is a right or even empowering response to the dilemmas raised by the decision and often necessity to manage human biology in science-based ways.

So what kind of a fact is death that it should remain open to such ongoing dispute? Brain death is no different from many other medical "facts"—it is as clear, and as vague, as the definition of asthma or high blood pressure. Death shares elements of ongoing uncertainty, contingency, and evolution that are true of most medical "facts." Ultimately, the value and resilience of such facts lie in how they fit together with other types of experience and in what these facts enable us to do when we use them. But the fact of brain death, as opposed to other facts, became caught up in debates over meaning that were fueled by the centuries-old awkwardness of describing human nature in terms of mind versus body. On the one hand, critics often found that the definition of brain death did not privilege the mind enough, arguing that the "higher" functions of consciousness should be the main criteria for human life and personhood and, consequently, that the loss of the higher functions should allow the declaration of brain death. On the other hand, the definition of brain death was just as often criticized for placing too much emphasis there, and so others argued that conflating life with a cognitive foundation to personhood naively ignored the fundamental biological life of the body. Debates in conferences and journals over how brain death was or wasn't justified therefore turned on questions of an unanswerable sort, such as: What is the meaning of identity? Questions like this elevated ethical or philosophical expertise about meanings over biological expertise about bodies as the driving consideration in how death should be defined.

How medical facts are established and used has great consequences. But the ethical framing of medical dilemmas, and especially the professionalization and formalization of ethics in healthcare settings, may have been more a symptom of—rather than the right solution for—an underdeveloped capacity for standardizing and brokering effective and affordable medical practices. The use of conceptual, ethical, and moral language about healthcare dilemmas can only go so far as a solution to this failure, and the story of brain death suggests that it did not go very far at all. An appeal, for example, to protect individual autonomy has been used for conservative and liberal political impulses alike, and as a rhetorical flourish to hide entrenched interests, or a genuine recourse to safeguard freedom and choice. That appeal, at the heart of the bioethical project, has had as much mixed cost and benefit in the medical context as it has in the political.

In the end, handwringing over carefully parsed meanings of personhood and autonomy proved clumsy tools to use to reach consensus over brain death in particular, and more generally over issues such as futility, medical necessity, and the aims of medicine. Not surprisingly, public discourse around issues ranging from Terry Schiavo to national healthcare reform descends into a spiral of morally charged but substantively impoverished accusations and finger-pointing about identity, rationing, religion, death panels, or socialism. The United States has the highest cost per citizen for healthcare of any country, but the least value to show for it; the United States also originated bioethics and turned it into an industry—a development whose value-add is also less than clear. The sprawling growth in medical technology and the simultaneous expansion of bioethics is no coincidence. The story of brain death underscores how moralizing the analysis of hard choices might work around, rather than directly address, problems we won't—or can't—confront very well.

These are not the conclusions or issues I started with when I began to research the origins of the brain death criteria. I was initially focused on what these pages mostly describe: the circumstances, evidence, and purposes that drove the appearance of brain death in the middle of the twentieth century.

NOTES

1.   Ad Hoc Committee of the Harvard Medical School to Examine the Definition of Brain Death, "A definition of irreversible coma," *Journal of the American Medical Association* 205, no. 6 (August 5, 1968): 337–40.

2. I will refer to "medicine," "medical practice," etc throughout this book. By "medicine," I generally mean common usage that describes the organized and applied use of human biological sciences to intervene and alter body functions in validated ways to treat or identify illness, and improve health. The focus of this study—brain death and hospital-based care—means attention is given to physician-professionals and more acute, specialized, care. I fully recognize and encourage broadening that applied use to include a range of actors beyond physicians, as well as to address health promotion goals beyond acute disease. However elastically one wishes to consider the scope of the term "medicine," the core points made here about sourcing values from medical knowledge still apply, and indeed are crucial to successfully broadening that scope.

3. Eelco F. M. Wijdicks, Panayiotis N. Varelas, Gary S. Gronseth, and David M. Greer, "Evidence-based guideline update: Determining brain death in adults. A Report of the Quality Standards Subcommittee of the American Academy of Neurology," *Neurology* 74 (2010): 1911–18; President's Commission on Ethical Problems in Medicine and Biomedical and Behavioral Research, *Defining Death: A Report on the Medical, Legal, and Ethical Issues in the Definition of Death* (Washington DC: US Government Printing Office, 1981); President's Council on Bioethics, *Controversies in the Determination of Death* (Washington DC: December 2008).

4. Joseph Fletcher, "Technological Devices in Medical Care," in *Who Shall Live? Medicine, Technology, Ethics,* ed. Kenneth Vaux (Philadelphia: Fortress Press, 1970), 116–42, 121.

5. Georges Canguilhem, *The Normal and the Pathological,* Carolyn R. Fawcett (trans) (Brooklyn, NY: Zone Books, 2007 [1964]).

6. Jonathon Moreno, *The Body Politic: The Battle over Science in America* (New York: Bellevue Literary Press, 2011).

7. Mary Poovey, *A History of the Modern Fact: Problems of Knowledge in the Sciences of Wealth and Society* (Chicago: University of Chicago Press, 1998), 96.

8. The technocratic role for bioethics in the context of the search for rules, especially around genetic research and interventions, is made in John H. Evans's *Playing God? Human Genetic Engineering and the Rationalization of Public Bioethical Debate* (Chicago: University of Chicago Press, 2002).

9. Gary S Belkin, "Toward a historical ethics," *Cambridge Quarterly of Healthcare Ethics,* 10 no. 3 (2001): 345–350; Gary S Belkin, Allan M Brandt, "Bioethics: using its historical and social context," *International Anesthesiology Clinics,* 39 no. 3 (Summer 2001): 1–11.

"Strange Business"

"I wonder if you and I could not write a very useful paper together, with some such title as THE RIGHT TO DIE...Our efforts can be a truly pioneering endeavor."

—HENRY BEECHER TO WILLIAM CURRAN, *June, 1967*

"It was a strange business...how do we know these people are dead?" remarked Robert Young, a neurologist who arrived at Massachusetts General Hospital (MGH) in the 1960s. He was recalling encounters with severely comatose and respirator-dependent patients who appeared on hospital floors with accelerating frequency beginning in the mid to late 1950s. At MGH, Young had a neurology fellowship with Robert Schwab. Among other accomplishments in neurology, Schwab developed what he referred to as his "triad," a set of clinical findings that formed the basis of the criteria found in the Report of the self-appointed Ad Hoc Committee of the Harvard Medical School to Examine the Definition of Brain Death, which appeared in the *Journal of the American Medical Association* on August 5, 1968.[1] During much of the time the Committee deliberated, Schwab was at home convalescing from a heart attack, so Young represented him at Committee meetings.

Young later recalled an odd discomfort when he approached a unique kind of comatose patient. There was something familiar in these bodies yet something foreign as well, a blurring of the signs that had reliably set the line between death and life. Eventually, that line would be restructured altogether. "And the fact is we do live in a time of transition," German theologian and ethicist Helmut Thielicke noted at a prominent early gathering of the nascent bioethics field, the 1969 Houston Conference on Ethics in Medicine and Technology. Thielicke continued, "Advances in man's technical and scientific capacity have outstripped, as it were, the development of man himself...What man 'can do' is out of step with what man 'is'...At what point does help cease to be help and begin to cancel itself out? Can it still be called 'help' when all that remains of the patient is a physical or mental torso?"[2]

These, of course, weren't the first or last patients to provoke hesitation and strange uncertainty over the gap between common, lived experience and the experience of being a medical subject or biological object. Long before the advent of respirators and the idea of brain death, determining the moment of death has been an ongoing source of apprehension and changing social ritual. As historian Martin Pernick notes, "There never was a Golden Age of Hearts and Lungs when defining death was unambiguous and certain."[3] However, the ability to choose to maintain the familiar, though malleable, signs of a moving heart and expanding lungs, and to keep the body "working" with respirators and other medical interventions, brought a new and far-reaching ambiguity to the end of life. Referring to sixteenth-century and seventeenth-century Parisian funerary practices, Vanessa Harding notes the enduring importance of the question: "For how long does the dead human body retain the meanings and values it held in life, once it no longer has an incumbent but is perceived by outsiders only?"[4] The appearance of severe coma challenged previous medical consensus and cultural practice as to where to draw this line between incumbency and objectivity; between objects and persons. It further highlighted the constant—and unavoidable—redrawing of that line through medical encounters.

The strangeness of the mechanically active, moving, pink, comatose body moved some in medicine to confidently render this body irreversibly comatose, and to go further and define this condition as irreversibly dead. "Our primary purpose is to define irreversible coma as a new criterion for death," declared the opening lines of Beecher's Report.[5] But even in this opening sentence, ambiguity undermines the certainty of Beecher's pronouncement.

A particular kind of coma—a term describing an illness or a treated impairment of the *living* body—became, at the same time, the sign of the *absence* of a living body and the end of treatment. Death could be named in some aspects before it existed in others. It could be deliberated over, *decided*. The appearance of a new world of "death before dying" was a highly significant development in the history of medicine. This new way of approaching death and the body—which began in specialized corners of medical practice and continues to migrate through and reinforce other developments in (at least much of Western) society at large—is central to the story of brain death and to the alternating resistance and accommodation to living in a biomedical culture.

The thirteen Ad Hoc Committee members were distinguished faculty of Harvard University; all but three—theologian Ralph Potter, attorney and legal medicine expert William J. Curran, and historian of science Everett Mendelsohn—were physicians at Harvard Medical School. The name of Henry K. Beecher, then the Henry Isaiah Dorr Professor of Research and Teaching in Anaesthetics and Anaesthesia at Harvard Medical School and Chairman of the Department of Anesthesiology at MGH, appeared with the title "chairman" in small type at the bottom of the first of four published pages. Following his name were listed those of the remaining twelve members, in alphabetical order.

The Report was the result of collective deliberations, significant edits, and the resolution of a few pointed disagreements. However, the Report was clearly Beecher's, and was set in motion with a presentation Beecher made as Chairman of the Harvard Medical School Standing Committee of Human Studies. "With your permission," Beecher wrote to then Medical School Dean Robert H. Ebert in a letter dated September 6, 1967, "I should like to call a meeting of the Standing Committee of Human Studies." He continued:

At this meeting I should like to present, roughly, a 25 or 30 minute discussion of ETHICAL PROBLEMS CREATED BY THE

HOPELESSLY UNCONSCIOUS PATIENT. As I am sure you are aware, the developments in resuscitative and supportive therapy have led to many desperate attempts to save the dying patient. Sometimes all that is needed is a decerebrated individual. These individuals are increasing in numbers all over the land and there are a number of problems which should be faced up to.[6]

Beecher wrote to future Ad Hoc Committee members such as his long-time friend Curran, a professor of health law at Harvard, and neuroscientist Jordi Folch-Pi, to insure they would attend this presentation.[7] Curran had received letters from Beecher just the previous June suggesting that they write a paper entitled "THE RIGHT TO DIE" in order to address the problem of needless care for persons whose "brain has ceased to function."[8] When Beecher wrote Curran, he specifically linked the idea of a right to die—an idea vaguely and variably present in leading medical and law journals—with the idea that the cessation of brain function was the physiologic equivalent of death itself:

In this paper I think we will have to face up to what death really is. The ancient idea that when the respiration stops and the heart stops, death ensues is perfectly true, but is it not also death when the brain has ceased to function, as indicated by the absence of electrical activity? All major hospitals are confronted with situations where at great cost, and really at the expense of salvageable individuals, occasionally decerebrated subjects use up the money probably better spent elsewhere.[9]

That presentation was quickly followed with an October 20, 1967 letter to transplant surgeon Joseph Murray of the Peter Brent Brigham Hospital (later renamed Brigham and Women's Hospital in Boston), also in attendance. Beecher underscored "how strongly I agree with you that it would be most desirable for a group at Harvard University to come to some subtle conclusion as to a new definition of death."[10]

Beecher used his October presentation, and in particular Murray's support and interest, to make a case to Ebert for a specific committee to consider "the idea of brain death."[11] Ebert agreed.[12] Beecher picked most of the members himself. He tapped Curran and also MGH colleagues Raymond Adams, who was Chairman of Neurology, and neurologist Robert Schwab. Jordi Folch-Pi, whom Beecher also sought out to attend his Human Studies presentation, was also included, as were famed MGH neurosurgeon William Sweet and Murray, who received the Nobel Prize for performing the first human kidney transplantation. Beecher sought several non-physicians, listing in his own notes historian of science Everett Mendelsohn and sociologist David Riesman, although the latter did not eventually serve on the Committee. Beecher very much wanted to include a theologian. He thought his friend Joseph Fletcher would be a strong asset, but Fletcher was too publicly (and, therefore, controversially) associated with advocacy for a right to euthanasia. Beecher eventually settled on Ralph Potter of the Harvard Divinity School. Ebert suggested rounding out the representation by Harvard hospitals, and psychiatrist Dana L. Farnsworth, physiologist Clifford Barger, and neurologist Derek Denny Brown were added.

The whole group—Adams, Barger, Curran, Brown, Farnsworth, Folch-Pi, Mendelsohn, Merrill, Murray, Potter, Schwab and Sweet—were addressed by Ebert in a January 4, 1968 letter appointing them as members:

> At a recent meeting of the Standing Committee on Human Studies, Dr. Henry K. Beecher reviewed some basic material on the ethical problems created by the hopelessly unconscious man. Dr. Beecher's presentation re-emphasized to me the necessity of giving further consideration to the definition of brain death.[13]

Notably, Ebert continued this letter, "As you are well aware, many of the ethical problems associated with transplantation and other developing areas of medicine hinge on appropriate definition. With its pioneering interest in organ transplantation, I believe the faculty of Harvard Medical School is better equipped to elucidate this area than any other single group. To this end I ask you to accept appointment to an *ad hoc* committee." Throughout the committee's work from March into June of

1968, several members wrote to Beecher stating strongly that they did not think they were solving a transplantation problem but a very different problem.[14] Ebert himself would later back off from the transplantation reference. When the Report of the Ad Hoc Committee was presented to him for the final revision before publication, Ebert requested only one change, indicating that perhaps the text "suggests that you wish to redefine death in order to make viable organs more readily available...Would it not be better to state the problem, and indicate that obsolete criteria for the definition of death can lead to controversy in obtaining organs for transplantation?"[15]

How do we understand this exchange? Was Ebert—and was the Report itself—expressing a wish to expedite, or instead to police transplantation? How central to the Committee's purposes was either task? The issue of transplantation surfaces early on in the story of the Committee and dominates historical characterizations of it later. Soon after Beecher made his presentation to his colleagues and his pitch to Ebert, the first human heart transplant was performed by Christiaan Barnard on December 3, 1967, in Capetown, South Africa. The medical and public press captured a flurry of similar attempts that followed worldwide, but media coverage soon shifted to convey a subsequent flurry of failures, opening questions as to the wisdom as well as the eerie transgressions of the procedure. Were heart donors dead if their hearts continued to live? What boundaries distinguished one person's life from another? What process would legitimize the procedure of donating organs?

The coma that would count as death by Beecher and his colleagues attracted increasing interest. As the Committee met, newspapers reported stories about transplant surgeons accused of causing, rather than intervening after, the deaths of comatose patients in order to obtain organs. Clearly, confusion on this score could prove a fatal obstacle to the new and still fragile field of transplantation—confusion that could presumably be resolved by a revised definition of death. Curran wrote to Beecher about three such cases that appeared in Houston hospitals and that raised the question as to whether a patient was dead before—or instead killed by—the removal of treatment and/or organs for the purposes of transplantation. Curran was concerned here that surgeons acted too hast-ily, demonstrating the possibility of "illegal and unethical conduct" and being "prematurely declared dead," suggesting that his remark to Beecher in this letter that "the issues we are talking about are not academic" was, regarding transplant, responding to an interest in policing its use. Other evidence will underscore this point, including the ways that transplant figured into the Committee members' respective life's work and input into the Report itself.[16]

The Committee's purposes with respect to transplant are important because of the prominent, consequential, but largely inaccurate uses made of these purposes by others, and the degree to which this inaccu-racy has closed off needed curiosity over how brain death *did* make sense as a solution to those who first formally defined it. Early critics of the committee doubted medicine's ability to follow Beecher in his pursuit to define the death of a patient, while at the same time reliably pursuing their "RIGHT[s]." Their accusations of stealth attempts to expand the scale of transplantation procedures underscored the case for changing who deter-mined medical ethics. This sort of characterization persisted in most his-torical descriptions of the Committee. Historian Tina Stevens' comments typify this vein of criticism:

> More than a medical response to a technologically-induced moral problem, "brain death" was an artifice of legal self-protection . . . against the possibility that the public would perceive a potential conflict of interest and become alarmed—a conflict between the profession's responsibility to care for the sick and dying and the demands of medical research to procure organs for transplant.[17]

Historical characterizations have generally taken this approach, tending to emphasize the Committee's efforts to expand transplantation practices and the associated inability of its members to grapple with the necessary philosophical and conceptual issues brain death posed. Critics further attribute these perceived tendencies to a lack of ethics expertise, arguing that Committee members were blinded by their immediate and "purely medical" purposes. Prominent voices and scholarship in bioethics have repeatedly toed this line. Portrayals of the Committee as transplantation-focused have carried the weight of a larger agenda, justifying the establishment of a distinct ethical expertise over medicine by bioethics. One influential example, Albert Jonsen's *The Birth of Bioethics*, found that the Report inadequately faced important philosophical questions about death in its overreaching and merely medical account. Jonsen contended that the argument for brain death was shallow in its science and ethics; cited no scientific data; and was a tool for grabbing organs for transplant.[18] In *Rethinking Life and Death*, Peter Singer suggested that the Committee was "not being entirely candid" by withholding the central role of transplantation in their deliberations.[19] Other prominent scholars of the history of brain death have argued that the Committee in fact hid its primary interest in transplants.[20] Few, if any, of these histories, however, engage the work of the Committee in detail.[21]

THE AUTHORS

For the key authors of the Report, *their* preoccupation was not with transplantation but with issues such as experimentation, truth-telling, and informed consent; the clinical signs of consciousness and coma; and the definitions and consequences of "hopeless" as well as "extraordinary" care. These are the topics that fill the following chapters of this book.

There were essentially three authors of the Report—Henry Beecher, Robert Schwab, and William Curran—with additional important input from Raymond Adams. The first meeting of the Committee, referred to in surviving minutes and drafts, was held on March 14, 1968. As the key players began to compose the Report, paper drafts and suggested edits circulated through Beecher's hands. The first full draft that appears in Beecher's files is dated April 11 of that year. Subsequent versions reviewed here are dated June 3, June 7, and June 13, with a final version dated June 25. The meeting schedule and correspondence in Beecher's papers show that most of the writing of the Report was done in bursts at the end of

April, and then again from the end of May into early June. The serial versions, along with the intervening correspondence and edits, indicate that the writing was primarily the work of Beecher, Schwab, and Curran, with some small refinements to the criteria themselves by Adams. Only weeks after completion, the paper appeared in print.

The April 11 draft outlines both the themes and the division of authorial labor that generally persisted throughout the Committee's work. Described as "a very preliminary draft of a report," the accompanying cover memo reported that "the legal section was, of course, written by Bill Curran, and the criteria of irreversible coma by Bob Schwab."[22] It is possible that the remaining documentary evidence leaves out other conversations and arguments that shaped the text. However, interviews and recollections with surviving Committee members confirm what the archival materials suggest: that Beecher essentially orchestrated the Report, pasting together written edits and contributions primarily from himself, Schwab, and Curran.

Beecher began working at MGH in the mid-1930s. At MGH, mentors encouraged him to change his plans to be a surgeon and instead to establish an academic program and laboratory science foundation for anesthesiology. When he assumed the Dorr Chair in 1941, the first endowed chair in anesthesiology in the world, he became an international leader in this field, helping to transform a then peripheral and poorly established medical specialty.[23] His research focused on the physiology and effectiveness of anesthetic agents and on the efficacy of medication for pain.

By the time the Report appeared, he had also published widely quoted work on the ethics of human experimentation, work that strongly shaped his thinking about irreversible coma. It is no accident that the Ad Hoc Committee to Examine Brain Death was, literally, an ad hoc committee of the Standing Committee on Human Studies at Harvard, which Beecher also chaired. Beecher wrote parts of his contributions for the Report long before the Ad Hoc Committee existed. He lectured and wrote about the problem of comatose patients raising questions about the limits of medical intrusiveness and the equitable and efficacious use of medical resources. Specific sentences and themes from these writings appeared in the Report.

The Report was his last significant project prior to retirement from MGH in 1969.[24]

Curran was a dominant figure in the development of the field of legal medicine through the latter twentieth century. He began teaching a series of interdisciplinary seminars on the interactions of law and medicine in the 1950s at Harvard Law School and the Harvard School of Public Health, and then went on to a position directing the Law-Medicine Research Institute at Boston University. He eventually returned to Harvard as a professor in the School of Public Health. After coming across some references of Beecher's, Curran began their relationship in 1958 with a letter to Beecher noting mutual interests.[25] The two engaged in a personal, and frequent, correspondence (Figures 1.1 and 1.2).

On the same day Beecher wrote Curran on the topic of "THE RIGHT TO DIE," a thirty-four-year-old alcoholic merchant marine, referred to as DM, collapsed and arrived unresponsive at MGH with bleeding on both sides of

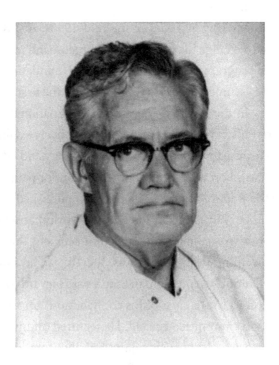

Figure 1.1 Henry K. Beecher (1904–1976).
SOURCE: Courtesy of Edward Lowenstein.

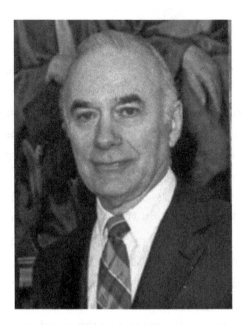

Figure 1.2 William J. Curran (1925–1996).
SOURCE: Courtesy of the President and
Fellows of Harvard College.

his brain. DM was unresponsive to pain and had no reflexes or spontaneous movement except for swallowing reflexes. He could breathe spontaneously but insufficiently on his own and required a respirator. Two electroencephalograms (EEGs or "brain wave" tests) obtained twenty-four hours apart were described by Schwab as "flat...with no distinguishable electrico-cortical activity." Based on his neurological status, DM's physicians informed his only adult family, his divorced wife, of the "grave prognosis," and an order was written to "D/C IV. No medications." Soon thereafter, DM died.[26]

DM was typical of the patients Schwab and his EEG laboratory staff encountered in consultation over the prior decade. EEG and physical examination findings were used to assess prognosis of severe brain injuries and to conclude whether removal of treatment seemed reasonable, if not compelling. DM did not fully meet Schwab's and the Committee's eventual criteria for brain death due to the preservation of a reflex in which the back of the throat, as gateway to the lungs, tightens or "gags" so as to prevent objects rather than just air from passing. He was also not apneic; that is, unable to mechanically initiate and sustain breaths on his own. But while he could generate respirations, these were insufficient to support life on their own. He was not "dead" but, without mechanical support, stood at death's threshold. It was through experience with hundreds of patients like DM that Schwab identified what seemed to him and colleagues with whom he consulted to describe the line between legitimate medical action and violation of a corpse.

Schwab closely matched Beecher in the timing of his arrival at and departure from MGH (Figure 1.3).[27] Accomplished in many areas—he established new treatments in myasthenia gravis and Parkinson's disease and was among the first to use dilantin for epilepsy—Schwab was an early user of EEG. In an obituary written by Young, he was described as having "founded the first clinical laboratory for the routine recording of electroencephalograms...in any part of the world, as far as is known."[28] Beginning at least in the 1940s, Schwab showed an interest in the fate of the EEG in determining human death. In a series of studies conducted throughout the 1960s he refined and defended what he called his "triad" of criteria—no movement or breathing, areflexia, and isoelectric, or "flat," EEG tracing—in order to clarify which symptoms or findings did and did not matter in establishing reliable outcome predictions for patients such as DM. This triad became the core of the Harvard criteria and of how brain death was then determined through much of the world.

Beecher was familiar with Schwab's work and advocated the use of his criteria before the Committee existed. Schwab had significant concerns about the implications of a more technologically intensive medicine for dignified death and dying, coauthoring, with Sidney Rosoff, a paper on his criteria that was cited in early drafts of the Report. Rosoff was a prominent leader in the US euthanasia movement in the 1950s and 1960s, serving on the boards and as president of both the Euthanasia Society of American and the Hemlock Society.[29]

These were the primary authors of the Report. Their sections and themes organize the next chapters of this book: *justification, law,* and *criteria.* These sections each reflect specific bodies of literature, histories,

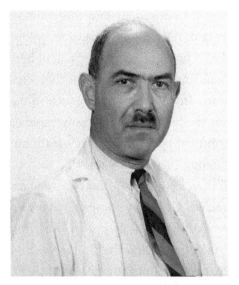

Figure 1.3 Robert Schwab (1903–1972).
SOURCE: Courtesy of Massachusetts General
Hospital Archives and Special Collections.

and cultures of practice. Revisiting these sources underscores how these authors were primarily motivated to address centuries-old questions about how to define the limits of medicine and medical necessity and how to use medical knowledge. Norms around practices like truth-telling and human experimentation were often drawn upon to provide possible answers to these questions. The strange coma, uncertainty, and manipulative power of conditions of death before dying made these questions more challenging and compelling. Especially for Beecher, brain death was a response to that challenge.

DEATH: A NEW PUZZLE

The appearance of positive-pressure adjunct lungs in the 1950s signaled a significant departure from decades of experience with the so-called "iron lung" used for polio patients since the 1930s. The iron lung tank was a cylinder that fully surrounded a person from the neck down and alternately evacuated and then reintroduced air into this cylinder. Reduction of air pressure within the tank relative to the outside, where the person's head remained, established a negative pressure gradient between the air accessible to the mouth and nose compared with that surrounding the chest within the iron lung. This alternating pressure difference enabled the chest walls, and thus the lungs, to more easily expand, enabling the person to inhale. Intermittent positive pressure breathing machines (IPPBs) replaced this technology in the 1950s. IPPBs instead forced air under "positive pressure" directly into the lungs in regular bursts via a tube inserted into the trachea. Generally, these machines also allowed patients who could breathe even weakly on their own either to do so, or to trigger the assistance of positive pressure as they initiated a breath. Design fundamentals have not changed significantly since.

The iron-lung substitute generally supported the breathing of someone fully conscious, for a usually limited period, during which time the poliovirus interfered with brainstem control over breathing or directly paralyzed muscles used for breathing.[30] If the patient survived this tenuous period, these viral effects on breathing soon remitted as the illness passed through its acute course. Like most hospitals, MGH relied on these devices as late as a polio epidemic in 1955.[31] The new IPPB respirators, however, could sustain more severe, less predictable, and longer-term impairment to breathing and began to be used beyond their initial role in the management of post-surgical, especially post-thoracic surgical, patients at MGH a few years later. Attention to IPPBs was spurred apparently by crude use of positive pressure systems (manually squeezing a bag to force air into a patient's lung through an inserted tube) at Danish hospitals during a polio epidemic there in 1952. But as indications for the use of IPPBs expanded to include a range of serious illness, so did the debilitating conditions with which patients were left after treatment. Hospital care now kept sicker people alive and left them in a more impaired state. Different costs and benefits began to line up against each other. Jack Emerson, who developed a widely used version of the iron lung in the 1930s, recalled how physicians often expressed concern that his new technology interfered with the natural course of illness and extended suffering. But such concerns were not commonly expressed. They did not play a significant role in the use of this technology.[32] The conditions of death before dying were only dimly, though at times presciently, perceived in the iron age:

> If the paralysis…should be permanent, we could not hope to accomplish anything. We would be forced to use the respirator indefinitely or until someone should turn executioner by stopping the machine, or until an intercurrent infection solved the problem for us.[33]

Eventually, however, concern about the limits and consequences of respirators eventually did grow alongside their expanded use. The new ambiguity of the body suspended and sustained by the respirator, and the expanded possibilities of intensive care medicine, prompted questions about the appropriateness of care and about physician identity as an intervener and risk manager.

This identity has an ongoing history. The consolidation of orthodox, or allopathic medicine practiced by licensed "mainstream" physicians came at the end of a busy nineteenth-century flurry of debates among a range of alternative, unlicensed, and variably educated groups of practitioners with competing schools of thought. This outcome is often attributed, especially by physicians, to key discoveries and related therapeutic successes around that time, such as identification of germs as the cause of disease. However, this is too simple an account. Much of the consolidation around the definition of the physician as a sanctioned expert guided by certain kinds of tested knowledge was, in retrospect, attractive for reasons other than the actual power of therapeutic knowledge at the time. This model of what a physician should be was "a cognitive system and a set of social practices"[34] that incorporated other social and institutional developments of the time, such as associations between progress and measurement, and the notion of quantification as an indication of objectivity and science.[35]

An asserted ability to provide discerning management of what historian Martin Pernick once described as a "calculus of suffering"—that is, to provide reliable counsel in navigating difficult trade-offs and decisions—was

particularly distinctive to this ascendant orthodoxy.[36] Pernick took
as the paradigmatic, if not specific, driver of this change the combination of promise and resistance that greeted the heralded—but also very
risky—surgical use of general anesthesia in 1846. As key features of
post-nineteenth-century health care, this recurring theme of describing
medical work through a scope of manipulation tempered through a testable
calculus is relevant for understanding much of the inherited vocabulary
and concerns that mattered to Committee members, especially Beecher.
The shifting meaning of the physician as "risk manager" describes a historical narrative that spans both early twentieth-century anxiety about
medical heroics and early twenty-first-century debates about the design
of health services. However completely or incompletely the "calculus of
suffering" narrative explains the emergence of a form of mid-to late nineteenth century medical practice and knowledge in the United States, it carries enduring relevance. It focuses attention on the capabilities of medical
knowledge, as well as the "cognitive system...and practice" within which
these capabilities worked. Compared to the prevailing rescue narrative of
bioethics, it directs curiosity to possible alignment between the capabilities of medical knowledge and concrete ways to frame and resolve medical
dilemmas. It also seems pertinent to the appearance of brain death and
the critical response to it. Beecher's experience of how this physician identity played out in the context of rapidly changing hospital-based medical
practices framed his thinking about brain death. That endurance should
get our attention.

STRANGE NEW WORLD

In an anonymously authored *Atlantic Monthly* article from 1957, which
indicated emerging alarm over medicine's ethic of preserving life at all
costs, a woman grieved the death of her husband:

There is a new way of dying today. It is the slow passage via modern
medicine. If you are very ill modern medicine can save you. If you are

going to die it can prevent you from doing so for a very long time…As they fight for spiritual release, and are constantly dragged back by modern medicine to try again, does their agony augment…Enter the sickroom and sit with your beloved, and endure the long watch while this incredible battle between spirit and medicine takes place.[37]

An editorial in the *New England Journal of Medicine* noted: "This is an article that cannot be summarized. It should be required reading for physicians." The editorial went on to argue that physicians should examine the effects of new medical technologies:

A decrease in dignity and rapport with the bereaved seems in inverse proportion to the efficacy of the medical sciences to prolong life. Perhaps there is no alternative, for certainly euthanasia is repugnant to every ideal of medical tradition. On the other side of the coin, however, is an approaching specter that looks almost as ghoulish and quite as menacing as euthanasia itself.[38]

The degree to which these anonymous remarks reflected broader public concern about the intrusiveness of medical technology is hard to gauge. Few articles like the *Atlantic Monthly* piece appeared over the following decade, and sporadic press attention to new medical technologies reflected a mixture of fascination and celebration, as well as anxiety. A more sustained and effective groundswell of concern does not appear until a flurry of newspaper editorials and special features appeared in response to the publication of the Harvard Report, further accelerated again by the Karen Ann Quinlan case when it was filed in 1975. Quinlan was a young, comatose woman whose parents wished to end medical treatment they saw as futile. The 1976 decision in that case by the Supreme Court of New Jersey recognized the legal standing of proxies to act for comatose patients and to authorize the removal of medical treatment. The publicity that surrounded this case mobilized public interest and attention around the value of intrusive, manipulative, and technologically intensive forms of therapy aimed at prolonging life.

The appearance of the Report, then, can be placed at the early outset of stronger public attention to these issues, including acceptance and humane treatment of terminal illness and renewed interest in euthanasia. By the 1970s, advocacy for euthanasia shed its beneficent, often eugenically oriented posture of earlier decades. Advocates instead framed euthanasia as more of a rights-based claim, an assertion of self-ownership over how people died or incorporated serious illness into their lives.[39]

But prior to these developments such issues were talked about in the medical literature, albeit hesitantly. In the early 1960s, articles began appearing in medical journals about what was often referred to as "the hopeless case," echoing a critique of medicine launched by Anonymous:

> In the last few years, I am sure many senior physicians (and some junior ones as well) have been troubled, as I have been, by certain of the effects of our increasing ability to prolong the life of people. The sulfonamides, the antibiotics, a better understanding of the uses of blood, machines such as artificial pacemakers, and artificial kidneys, the newer breathing apparatuses, radical and improved surgical techniques, our better knowledge of nutrition, etc. all have played a role at one time or another in saving, and hence prolonging the life of many people [but perhaps only prolonging suffering] . . . Who among us, after such sights can be proud of what we have wrought?[40]

Quoting with sympathy and agreement the remarks of Anonymous, Frank J. Ayd, a psychiatrist and a friend of Beecher's, argued in a 1962 lead article in *JAMA* that treating the terminally ill risked a situation in which "life preserving treatment ceases to be a gift and becomes instead, a scientific weapon for the prolongation of agony."[41] He strongly advocated for and elaborated on Papal endorsement of discontinuing extraordinary treatments:

> Since an individual has the right to dispose of his own person and, therefore, to have a voice in his manner of dying, he may not only

refuse extraordinary means of prolonging life, but he may also reject means which are ordinary but artificial and which offer no hope of a cure.[42]

Patient or family authorization of removal of care was not an uncommon practice. But it also does not appear to have been widespread. Papers and editorials in journals and medical newsletters indicate other activity, mentioning conferences, speeches at local symposia, and medical society meetings with panels of clergy, citizens, and physicians—all hard to enumerate and catalogue but signaling, nevertheless, interest and anxiety within the profession as to the nature of physician responsibility to not treat or to stop treating.

These traces of conversations about medical overreach within the profession highlighted two key considerations in defining the appropriateness of treatment. One was whether a patient's death occurring after a decision to withhold treatment was due to the inevitable course of disease in the face of passive omission or was, instead, the result of physician action—that is, of active commission. Another was the related difference between treatments considered to be "ordinary" versus those considered to be "extraordinary." The distinction between an illness that was allowed to meet its natural end as opposed to one that still compelled medical intervention had long been used to guide care of the very sick. The balance between ending treatment but not euthanizing—of being clear when one was permitting, and not causing, death—was a preoccupation of much of 1950s and 1960s literature on hopeless and futile cases, as it had been decades before and as it would remain decades later. Similarly, opinion as to which set of circumstances more convincingly cast an intervention as "ordinary" instead of "extraordinary" had long played a defining role in shaping consensus over what constituted acceptable care. For those with severe coma, much of the work of Schwab and other neurologists would involve describing how it was possible to know which signs described a treatable condition. More than simple prognosis was at stake in this calculus. Attempts to specify what fell outside of the "ordinary" also often drove an understanding of how (and whether) uncertain medical knowledge progressed. After all, how did, or does, medicine progress other than by constantly making the extraordinary, ordinary?

The implications of differentiating between ordinary and extraordinary treatment had been pondered since at least the nineteenth century: administration of oxygen to a patient who was breathing spontaneously (before the advent of respirators) but in a presumed irreversible coma; continued insulin treatment for a diabetic patient with terminal, painful, metastatic cancer; use of caffeine for a lethargic dying patient; the intense pains of necessary amputation; the use of general anesthesia at all. For each of these examples, sources could be cited which considered these extraordinary treatments.[43]

New ambiguity over when death occurred complicated how doctors were to make these distinctions between ordinary and extraordinary care, and between omission and commission of harm. That ambiguity needed to be addressed, and growing unease over when death occurred can be read in medical journals especially in the latter part of the 1960s.[44] This context, in which action versus omission and ordinary versus extreme care framed a calculus of suffering, helps understand (as will be discussed in more detail) the tension in the Report itself over why this seemingly new coma should not just describe when to end treatment, but how to define death. These new coma patients, supported by respirators and other new life-support technologies, seemed to blur these distinctions. One *JAMA* article remarked:

> I remember when cessation of heartbeat was an observation on which we simply pronounced the patient dead; now this is a medical syndrome known as cardiac arrest, which demands prompt, skilled, and at times heroic treatment...I have seen patients with brain-stem failure, with dilated, fixed pupils, decerebrate rigidity, and cessation of spontaneous respiration, who...were assisted with a mechanical ventilator...I have never seen such a patient begin to breathe spontaneously and survive, and autopsy always shows advanced liquefaction necrosis of the brain...When did the soul leave the body? Is turning off the respirator murder?[45]

"What and when is death?" read another *JAMA* editorial appearing in early May 1968, months before Beecher's Report.[46] The editorial responded to a paper in that issue of *JAMA* written by thoracic surgeon and attorney Martin Halley, and a teacher of his in law school, William F. Harvey, which pointed to the "serious difficulties sometimes encountered in establishing the end point of human existence, or moment of death, by present medical definitions and with use of available objective standards and current criteria."[47] Medical practices, they argued, were beginning to incorporate a new working understanding of death that the law needed to acknowledge. Life could no longer be reliably understood by the appearance of "vital functions" such as pulse and respirations, unless one meant the vital functions without artifice, without "extraordinary measures"—a definition supported by Pope Pius XII in an address to the International Congress of Anesthesiology, which met in Rome in 1957 and which Beecher himself took part in. While ceding to other experts the question of whether to define *death* as the cessation of brain function, the Pope had clear opinions about *extraordinariness*. "In those that are considered to be completely hopeless...it cannot be held that there is an obligation to use resuscitative interventions," nor was there an obstacle in the way of "letting the doctor remove the artificial apparatus before the blood circulation has come to a complete stop."[48]

Halley and Harvey identified a new level of complexity in the oft-used distinction drawn between treatments that were ordinary and those that were extraordinary. Use of "extraordinary" generally meant "uncommon," "experimental," or "unnatural" aspects of medical *practice*, but Halley and Harvey used extraordinary to describe the *condition* of some patients. What now became strange, or extraordinary, was the notion of death itself. The machinations of the intensive care unit (ICU) obscured and ended unmediated access to "ordinary" death.[49] Death before dying was strange business. "The concern was basically that there was a finite event that the patient was seen as alive, and then when you did something it was no longer alive...it wasn't seen as a withdrawal...That took some time to develop."[50]

This developing calculus of suffering applied old tools of omission and ordinariness to these new circumstances. These tools tended to underscore a certain understanding of medical knowledge with which they were aligned. They focused on the consequences, and therefore responsibilities, of physician judgment, and so were linked to attitudes that acknowledged but generally sidelined the patient's role as arbiter over decisions to pursue or withhold medical interventions. In a widely read article in *CA*, the American Cancer Society's informational journal for physicians involved in cancer treatment, entitled, "You are standing at the bedside of a patient dying of untreatable cancer," Mayo Clinic physician Edward Rynearson advocated for an end to the prolonged suffering caused by prolonged treatment and for listening to patient wishes to guide such decisions.[51] His article is of particular interest because of the response to it. Months later, *CA* editors published forty responses by physicians throughout the United States as well as other countries, including senior cancer practitioners, medical school professors, department chairs, deans, and American Cancer Society leaders. Of these forty, five respondents criticized and thirty-five generally supported Rynearson's sentiments as to the dangers of overreach. However, only five responses could be interpreted as explicitly supporting reliance on patient choice in drawing that line. Rynearson's critics and sympathizers alike voiced the perception that "most" physicians, patients, and people at large were of the opinion that physicians should withhold treatment to sufferers for whom treatment only delayed death.

This sort of response recurs throughout the medical literature, in which questions of what counted as "unremediable" suffering, and when treatment "only delayed death," tended to be answered by falling back on the notion of the skilled physician as risk-calculator rather than by leaving such judgments to the discretion of patient choice, which was perceived as potentially unreliable and ambiguous. Hahnemann Dean Charles Cameron wrote that his school would no longer subscribe to *CA* and took steps to insure its students would not even see the issue containing Rynearson's article:

> For ten years, while I was Medical and Scientific Director of the American Cancer Society, I fought for the philosophy of fighting for the life of the cancer patient up to the end and I did this in an effort to overcome the resignation and inertia which seemed to characterize the care of the

cancer patient in his last weeks. I do not know who is wise enough to say
what cancer is treatable, or when it becomes treatable. Certainly, many
cancers which we are treating today with a good deal of vigor and with
an immense amount of psychological and physical support to the patient
were considered untreatable at the time I was an intern.[52]

Subsequent generations of physicians, bioethicists, and judges would
argue that the patient was by necessity wise enough. But from the 1940s
well into the 1960s, physician commentaries on hopelessness, extraordinariness, and withholding treatment linked these themes together primarily through a shared focus on the perceived consequences of physician
abdication of responsibility for hard choices. A diminished commitment
to treating the severely ill would lead to neglected, "narcotized" victims
of therapeutic pessimism, slackened attention to advancing therapies,
illusory confidence in the certainty of prognoses, and the abandonment
of hope. As a result of these fears, even those who advocated for limited
treatment were not committed to full-bore patient autonomy.

This hesitant embrace for patient prerogatives by physicians can be,
and certainly has been, criticized as undermining claims physicians might
make as appropriate guarantors of medical ethics. But this criticism has
often also closed off curiosity about the issues of medical knowledge, purpose and progress that did preoccupy these physicians and that lay behind
much of this hesitation. The challenges of creating and using medical
knowledge underlay the longevity and usefulness of tests of ordinariness
and omission in medical dilemmas,, and shaped beliefs about how and
when to include patient prerogatives. Beecher understood these challenges in ways that informed how he considered this new coma to signal
not only the end of care, but the end of life.

BEFORE THE HOPELESS CASE: THE "RADICAL" CURE

Before the respirator and the ICU, the treatment of cancer raised questions of when and if treatment of disease was excessive. When was "radical

surgery" too radical? The dilemma was that improvement in complex surgical procedures required learning by first doing these procedures poorly,
thus potentially blurring the distinction between accepted treatment and
experiment. Only continued attempts at risky treatment could inform
progress and achieve greater success. This reverse Faustian bargain—hell
first, then possibly heaven in return—proved an exceptional calculus of
suffering and so, predictably, physicians tended to claim that its hazards
demanded exceptional professional integrity, beneficent motive, and technical excellence.

Improvements in surgical technique and postoperative management in
the 1940s and 1950s renewed surgical adventurism toward cancer along
with a related tendency to see medical progress as a series of hard choices.
Some radical abdominal resection surgeries for cancer showed surgical
mortality rates of 30 percent, with a similar probability of only achieving
palliation of symptoms in then end. In the context of other options, these
outcomes were considered encouraging signs, confirming the wisdom of
"a more radical attitude in regard to the surgical treatment of advanced
abdominal cancer."[53] There were few perceived alternatives to surgery for
cancer at this time. Surgeons could tangibly intervene in a dread disease at
a time when radiation or chemotherapeutic treatments were less effective,
even for palliation of symptoms. After all, "what are you going to do for
a patient who is so uncomfortable that she is a morphine addict?" asked
one of the leading gynecologic surgeons of his day, Joe Meigs of MGH.[54]
Many prominent surgeons—George T. Pack, Alexander Brunschwing,
and Jerome Urban at Memorial Sloan-Kettering in New York, Owen
H. Wangensten at the University of Minnesota, among them—proudly
promised ever more extensive surgical resection of cancer.[55]

In contrast, Harvey B. Stone, one of the more prominent critics of what
he called a "newer radicalism of cancer surgery," argued that it did not necessarily follow that just "because it is *possible* to do certain extensive operations…it is therefore sensible or desirable to do them." But at the same
time he observed that "we must see human progress equally dependent
on the sturdy retention of the proved good, and the adventurous search
for the unknown better."[56] His was a characteristic belief that management

of the relationship between risky treatment and progress was a defining feature of physicians. That experience of how medicine learned and progressed to improve outcomes was tightly connected to what physicians thought they owed those they treated in terms of disclosure, listening, and discussion of treatment options.

TRUTH-TELLING

"A major problem in managing the 'hopeless case' concerns the imparting of pertinent diagnostic and prognostic information to the patient," explained one early 1960s commentary.[57] The removal of large amounts of intestine, or half of someone's pelvis, carried significant surgical risk of mortality or disability; the possibility of a cure was uncertain and usually unlikely. Enormous costs mixed with the enormous uncertainty of benefit:

> Should all the possibilities in every case be outlined to the patient and then the burden of decision placed on him? Such decisions require perspective that the physician cannot often impart, even to the intelligent and emotionally well-balanced patient. Should the physician then become the personal advisor...? If [so], according to what norms...should he make this decision...[as] his manner of presentation will often be decisive in selection of therapy.[58]

Whether decision making was imposed or shared, neither choice, in this view, circumvented the ultimate responsibility of the physician to shape the course of treatment. While data that could help guide decisions for cancer surgery accumulated, it remained limited. The uncertainties these decisions presented were substantial and not resolved by passing responsibility for decisions on to patients, many physicians argued. The physician ultimately, unavoidably, needed to exercise judgment. While paternalism and professional authority is at work here, so is the management of uncertainty that Pernick placed at the center of medical knowledge, purpose, and identity.

A discussion in medical journals throughout 1950s and into the 1960s on the responsibilities and meanings of sharing "truth" with patients often boiled down more specifically to the question: Should the *cancer* patient be told? This question was perhaps the most written-about ethical issue during this period, with the possible exception of closely related questions about human experimentation. It also was perhaps one of the first empirically studied medical ethics issues. Donald Oken's frequently cited 1961 survey appeared at the end of a decade that included several published inquiries in surgery and cancer journals into physician practices and patient attitudes toward truth-telling about cancer diagnoses.[59] Despite the fact that an overwhelming majority of patients surveyed during this period expressed expectations of a truthful diagnosis, with only a significant minority expressing resistance or uncertainty over the idea,[60] the reported behavior of surveyed physicians generally showed more definitive resistance. Oken concluded that physicians relied on pat assumptions to explain their reticence to fully disclose this diagnosis; often, these assumptions weren't substantiated by their own reported experience, including, for example, the assumption that patients would be suicidal if clearly told they had cancer. The reason Oken offered for this was their own discomfort and fear of cancer and death. While physicians wished to be told about cancer when it came to their own diagnoses, they were generally fatalistic about the disease and delayed pursuit of its diagnosis when they had symptoms themselves.[61]

Oken's findings reflected a growing attention within medicine on the psychological dimensions of cancer treatment and the dynamics of medical decision making.[62] During this time, Oken was the Assistant Director of the Institute for Psychosomatic and Psychiatric Research and Training at the Michael Reese Hospital and Medical Center in Chicago, and his work reflected that of a slowly growing group of physicians interested in the study of the psychological well-being of patients facing serious illness. Michael Reese—a storied public hospital that closed in 2009 and was founded by Jewish immigrants in the impoverished south side of Chicago in the latter nineteenth century to serve all those in need of care—was home to the Institute, which was led by Roy Grinker. Grinker was trained in neurology as well as psychoanalysis as an analysand of Sigmund Freud.

He is credited with developing the "biopsychosocial" integrated model of disease and positioned the Institute, in its heyday, as a leader in efforts to re-describe psychological care in more integrated ways.

The growing presence of psychiatrists in medical hospitals through the middle of the twentieth century was fueled to a large degree by this interest in the psychological components of medical illness. These physicians sought empirical support for the relevance of the psychiatric and emotional dimensions of patient experiences with cancer and other illness, and studied long-assumed beliefs about the emotional impact of the information physicians gave cancer patients about their condition. Before the hospice movement and the emergence of routinely available care alternatives for the terminally ill, clinician investigators began to flesh out the principles of psychologically sensitive care for the dying and seriously ill, and produced a visible public literature that opened up the subject to larger attention.[63]

Arthur Sutherland, at Memorial Hospital in New York, and Jacob Finesinger, at MGH, used a detailed patient interview format to explore the psychological impact, resilience, and needs of cancer patients.[64] This work generally did not offer spirited advocacy for a specific obligation to tell—and an inherent right to hear—the full truth. But it did capture, in significant detail and poignancy, the burdens of disease and its treatment on individuals and their families.

This curiosity about illness experience tended to reinforce but also modify physician-driven prerogatives:

> "Good doctor–patient communication does not mean that the doctor give extensive lectures of frightening facts and statistics, but rather that he create an atmosphere in which the patient is encouraged to talk constructively about his problems... While the physician should not be evasive, he should certainly be circumspect in his direct statements. The physician should remember that the patient hopes more to be reassured than to be educated in oncology.[65]

While it was best to get the truth out there, it was generally advised to dole it out in portions for which the patient was deemed ready.[66] One frequently

quoted advocate of disclosure, the physiologist and clinical researcher
Walter C. Alvarez, wrote that "medical lying is wrong, usually futile, and
even harmful." He was, nonetheless, a critic of "lying" in degree, not kind.
He explained, for example, that if he found inoperable prostate cancer in an
elderly man, especially if that man had concurrent heart disease or hypertension that probabilistically could kill him first, the patient would not be
burdened with this information. "[T]he physician should talk or keep silent,
depending on the patient's courage and willingness to hear the truth."[67]

Psychiatric advice also emphasized that physicians needed to face their
own fears,[68] as well as appreciate the psychological strategies used by those
facing serious illness, so that they could be more engaged and responsive
but still, necessarily, remain the primary decision makers: "Questionnaires
and moralistic generalizations about 'always' telling or not telling a
patient...are of little value in helping a particular patient who is faced
with the problem not as an abstract question but as an agonizing immedi-
acy."[69] This seemingly mixed message—to make highly edited disclosures
but also assert full commitments to patients—was compelling at the time
in the way it called upon the longstanding belief that the expertise of physicians lay in the application of medical knowledge to particular persons,
along with the responsibility to weigh interventions against the costs specific to each person: "A policy [with regards to truth telling] implies uniformity and uniformity is a distillate of indolence and insensitivity having
no place in the practice of medicine."[70]

John Gregory's groundbreaking eighteenth-century treatise on medical
ethics reads almost the same way.[71] His discussion of truth-telling sorts
through clues as to the impact and imperfections of prognosis, but it also
unfolds within another argument. That argument was to convince readers
that the way he talked about knowledge and professionalism was a break
from prior uses of knowledge that were anchored more in social position
than in expertise and science. In this way his self-description as applying
knowledge with patients as a "gentleman" might sound quaint and conde-
scending to our ears but was radical and provocative to those of his contemporaries. His account captured a larger social change in Britain where
natural knowledge and scientific work reinforced a revised social order.[72]

Then, and again in the United States centuries later, information was itself considered a potential therapy, or danger. More than just emotional awkwardness or simple professional power was at stake in how physicians disclosed information. Across centuries then, debate and advice about truth-telling practices reflected differing commitments to the nature of medical knowledge, certainty, and physician role, and were situated within a broader cultural milieu and norms of disclosure.[73] Should the cancer patient be told the truth? Articles and books addressing this question from the 1950s through the late 1960s advised doing so. That inclination, however, was heavily qualified by the calculations of patient "benefits" and "risks" within a contingent and otherwise overwhelming mix of sickness, hope, and suffering.[74]

Of course, the extent to which such committed and beneficent relationships were actually practiced and experienced cannot be determined from this literature. There has been limited, careful study of the nature of doctor–patient interactions directly through patient diaries, letters, or medical records for example. Conceit, condescension, and bias are palpable in this truth-telling literature to be sure. But the emergence of a vocabulary for incorporating the reality of care for people, and the airing of otherwise previously quiet subjects, is evident as well: detailed descriptions of painfully held beliefs by some cancer patients, such as notions that they caused their cancer by moral or sexual transgression. Other examples of emerging disclosure were found in the experiences of women, especially those with hysterectomies or mastectomies who faced isolation wrought from their own (and their spouse's) resentments of mutilated sexuality and impaired domestic roles. Still other patients spoke of debilitating depression and anxiety associated with the cancer diagnosis when faced with inadequate support, intervention, and/or information from the physician. Published case studies and anecdotes, the dread and discomfort palpable in both public and medical sources, and references in medical accounts attesting to the variability in patient preference for information perhaps reflected some greater ambivalence and fear about truth by patients than surveys suggested. The public in many ways shared and fueled reaction to cancer as a dread disease, as well.[75] Answering the dilemmas of intrusive

medicine by simply trying to raise the voices of patients and diminishing those of physicians in later decades did not necessarily solve the
deeper challenge that animated prior centuries of physician approaches
to truth-telling: discerning which medical evidence matters and how to
incorporate and satisfy both the sufferer's subjectivity and application of
objectivity in the medical encounter and in healing practices that rest on
biology.

After the 1960s, challenging beneficence as a cornerstone of that dis-
cernment and instead centering decision-making in patients required,
argued critics, cracking open what Jay Katz described in the title of his
1984 book as "the silent world of doctor and patient."[76] That book and
that characterization have proved to be highly influential in shaping a historical picture of prior physician practices with respect to truth-telling
and informed consent that required the forceful crowbar of other experts
to open up and challenge. Two legal cases in particular are cited as the
leading edge of such disruption to the silence; *Salgo v. Leland Stanford,
Jr. University Board of Trustees*, in 1957, and *Natanson vs. Kline* in 1960.[77]
The first earned Katz's distinction as the first light shed upon that closed
world. Yet a reading of both opinions, and of legal writing about them
at the time, suggests more complex shifts. Indeed, these and other court
rulings well into the 1960s continued to support the idea that appropriate
disclosure included physician judgments about what patients were ready
to, or needed to, hear. While *Salgo* pronounced that a physician violated
duty to a patient by withholding facts necessary for "intelligent consent,"
that case was described by a contemporary judicial ruling as reflecting
an "extreme view."[78] Other jurisdictions soon before and after *Salgo* or
Natanson argued the more sustained point of view (up to this time) that,
for example, failure to disclose out of fear of causing excessive duress to
patients "cannot be deemed such want of ordinary care as to import liability."[79] Specifically, failure to disclose risk of laryngeal nerve damage in an
operation needed to be understood in the following way:

> Doctors frequently tailor the extent of their pre-operative warnings
> to the particular patient, and with this I can find no fault. Not only is

much of the risk of a technical nature beyond the patient's technical understanding, but the anxiety, apprehension, and fear generated by full disclosure thereof may have a very detrimental effect on some patients.[80]

Such privileging of physician discretion and attention to emotional reaction was common. Even *Natanson,* hailed as a groundbreaking precedent in revealing and cracking the code of silence, endorsed this background consensus with respect to truth-telling. *Natanson* involved a claim for damages for injuries sustained from cobalt radiation treatment. The Supreme Court of Kansas ruled on the narrow issue of whether conditions existed to re-try the case. The Court agreed that there were inadequate jury instructions as to whether any liability attributed to hospital personnel applied as well to their supervisory physician. In the course of reviewing the case, the court commented:

> There is probably a privilege, on therapeutic grounds, to withhold the specific diagnosis where the disclosure of cancer or some other dread disease would seriously jeopardize the recovery.[81]

The court also pointed out that *Salgo's* initial instruction that a physician disclose all facts affecting his "rights and interests and of the surgical risk, hazard and danger, if any" was found on appeal to be overly broad, and the reviewing court cautioned of the need to "recognize that each patient presents a separate problem, that the patient's mental and emotional condition is important and in certain cases may be crucial..."[82]

So, with respect to physician disclosure and informed consent, degrees of truth-telling, the ideal of physician-as-balancer, and the perceived role of the physician as emotional gatekeeper of information were connected in legal reasoning as well as in medical journals, conferences, and practices. Furthermore, subsequent changes in acceptable practice and legal standards were patchy and inconsistently applied or understood. At the time they were issued, rulings like *Salgo* and *Natanson* were not obviously headed in the directions that bioethicist commentators later attributed to them—a direction that some legal scholar contemporaries of Beecher and Curran warned these decisions were mistakenly construed to imply.[83]

That is not to question the path since these rulings toward patient participation in receiving and weighing medical information but rather to emphasize that it was a long path, remains a work in progress, and still succeeds or fails to the degree it is in dialogue with the conditions in which medical facts work. Pursuit of participatory, co-created, medical knowledge has recurred ever since there has been writing about healing. The debates over brain death after the Report appeared will illustrate the challenges of moving from participatory form and aspiration, to participatory content and realization. Successful participatory and patient-centered care even more so requires being curious to learn and take into account what medical facts can do, how they work, and how they are generated.

EXPERIMENT

In addition to omission, ordinariness, and truth-telling, another key set of understandings that Beecher drew upon, described further in the next chapter, was expectations surrounding ethical experimentation. Setting clear rules around human experimentation is usually timed by ethicists and historians to follow WWII, the investigation of Nazi uses of humans in research, and the subsequent Nuremberg Code, which resulted from the prosecution of some of the Nazi medical leadership charged with responsibility. While it is difficult to make broad generalizations about the general conduct of research in the postwar decades, there was clearly widespread interest in the issue of human experimentation ethics. Irving Ladimer's 1963 anthology of papers on human experimentation included excerpts of seventy-three papers written primarily in the previous decade, with an accompanying bibliography exceeding five hundred citations of English literature.[84]

Historical characterizations of debates over experimentation ethics tend to portray the Nuremberg Trial prosecutions and the resulting Code as the start of a line of thinking that replaced physician judgment, with patient choice. That line of thinking, and the path it took, was far from straightforward, however. How and why did physicians concerned about experimentation ethics discuss Nuremberg? Why did they, and other non-physician commentators, generally consider research ethics to be best understood, again, as a product of physician integrity, beneficence, and prerogative? Delving into these questions complicates a history that posits the straightforward movement of patient-choice principles out of Nuremburg.

The so-called "Code" of Nuremberg was, more specifically, a section in the published judgment of the trial which took the form of a list of ten characteristics of "Permissible Medical Experiments" culled by the presiding judges from the unspecified consensus of "protagonists of the practice of human experimentation."[85] The American Medical Association (AMA) sent physician and physiologist Andrew C. Ivy as a medical expert to the team prosecuting Nazi physicians. Along with a draft of principles penned by another expert witness, neurologist Leo Alexander, Ivy, in his report to the AMA, apparently generated much of the language used by the Nuremberg judges in writing the Code.[86] For Ivy these rules were, as the Court's opinion implied them to be, "well established by custom, social usage and the ethics of medical conduct,"[87] and reflected a "common understanding."[88]

The opinion responded to the defense assertion that these doctors technically met expectations of proper conduct because, as they argued, the subjects after all gave "consent." Subjects purportedly consented since they were given the chance, for example, for a reprieve from a death sentence in exchange for research participation. No surprise, then, that the Code elaborated in exhaustive detail that *uncoerced* informed consent is required from the subject. The detail was tailored to close off creative loopholes— offered at trial by the defense—by thoroughly describing expectations that were "well established by custom."

The authors of the Code had more immediate objectives than to explicate an ethical theory of informed consent to replace physician virtue and beneficence. From the published proceedings and histories of both Alexander's and Ivy's contributions, it seems more plausible to argue that the Court's motivation was to reinforce those virtues. The Court reacted to the sheer horror at the brutality of these experiments by people who were trusted to have known better. The experiments struck those who judged them as, essentially, an abandonment of the kind of relationship and fidelity doctors were expected to owe patients—be they recipients of treatment or research—all in order to service the needs of a racist state and conform to a vile political culture. As historian of Nazi medicine Robert Proctor has noted, "The [Nazi] doctors...were not morally blind or devoid of the power of moral reflection...the primary failing of Nazi medicine, I would argue, was the failure of physicians to challenge the rotten, substantive core of *Nazi* values."[89] Yale law professor Robert Burt discouraged investing in Nuremberg the origins of a trans-historical ideal of patient/subject self-determination. The Code was instead a historically specific response. Investing the Nuremberg decision with these other meanings was a later development.[90]

For decades following WWII, physicians who described the proper conduct of experiments built upon a pre-WWII emphasis to distinguish between research that was therapeutic (research that was aimed at testing treatment for a patient) versus research that was nontherapeutic (research primarily aimed at collecting information of scientific interest without a prospect of benefit to that patient). Since the early twentieth century, this therapeutic/nontherapeutic distinction was a central concept for policing whether an experiment was proper or not and for determining how medical organizations, such as the AMA and medical school faculties, reconciled a growing commitment to organized research as still part of a physician's core therapeutic identity.[91] Defining most research as therapeutic legitimated it within the usual physician exercise of ordinary care. The traditional therapeutic/nontherapeutic distinction could help guard against a threat highlighted by the Nazi and Nuremberg experiences—loss of the proper balance between pursuit of obligations to patients and pursuit of obligations or benefits to society.

This logic was evident in much of the literature on experimentation ethics in the mid to late twentieth century. The inherent difficulties of achieving adequate informed consent, and of subjects truly grasping and investigators fully specifying the complexities and unknowns of an experiment—after all, by definition experiments involve risks and benefits that cannot be reliably known—were widely discussed. Some argued that if the risks of a nontherapeutic experiment were likely inconsequential, then it could be conducted without consent. Codes of experimentation ethics proliferated through the 1960s, including those of the British Medical Research Council (1963, [1953]), the British Medical Association (1963), the World Medical Association (Helsinki Declaration, 1964), and the American Medical Association (1966).[92] All these simplified the more expansive Nuremberg definition of informed consent and explicitly required it only of nontherapeutic, and not therapeutic, research. Actually achieving the level of communication and understanding detailed in this much-discussed first item of the Code was thought by skeptics to be infeasible.[93]

It is hardly surprising that physicians defended idealized norms of beneficent medical practice as better protection for individuals against the possible dangers of research. But others argued this as well. Philosopher Samuel Stumpf, in a paper described by early bioethicist Albert Jonsen as the "first philosophical contribution to medical ethics," found consent both morally indecisive (could one be permitted to consent to *anything*?) and often not feasible.[94] The more skepticism a particular writer had about the reliability of consent, the more their ethical standard for acceptable research rested on the degree to which a study mirrored usual physician beneficent responsibilities in ordinary care.[95] The more an experiment replicated the uncertainties considered common to routine care, the more usual physician leeway over disclosure in regular practice was considered adequate for research as well.[96] The Nazi experience seemed only to reinforce the view that human subjects were best protected by the usual practices of ordinary medicine, policed by the beneficent ethic of that enterprise. This general understanding considered likelihood of abuse of subjects to be greatest in the absence of the guiding goal of benefit. On this score, some physicians voiced concern about Nuremburg's *permissiveness* in sacrificing the individual for public gain.[97]

MEDICAL KNOWLEDGE, MEDICAL ETHICS

Parsing expectations of disclosure along degrees of therapeutic versus nontherapeutic purpose reflected an attitude about medical knowledge that included therapeutic "experimenting" within the scope of normal medical practice. That attitude was opposed to setting researcher and clinician identity farther apart from each other —a dichotomy which, as the Nazi experience also seemed to make clear, had to be avoided.[98] The link between the Nazi experience and the need to clarify therapeutic and nontherapeutic responsibilities was frequently made explicit.

The legal literature on human experimentation mirrored much of what physicians were saying in this regard. A prominent Yale Medical Society panel discussion of the Nuremberg Code highlighted this tension:

> Every doctor in the course of his daily practice engages in the conduct of experiment with his patients... the kind of clinical investigation which is more in the realm of pure scientific endeavor... where the information obtained is not likely to be of immediate value to the subject of the experiment... [Here is] the nub of our question.[99]

Ladimer was one of the most prolific commentators on the legal aspects of experimentation in the 1950s and 1960s. He was a faculty member of the Law-Medicine Research Institute at Boston University, founded in 1958 by William Curran, Beecher's friend and fellow Ad Hoc Committee member. Both Ladimer and Curran acknowledged repeatedly what the clinical literature anxiously observed—that there was no clear statutory or jurisprudential understanding of experiment as a legal activity. "Experiment" generally referred, since eighteenth-century English common law cases, to the deviation by physicians from accepted treatments. Physicians, this tradition emphasized, deviated from accepted practice "at their peril." Mid-twentieth-century physicians, especially in the shadow of Nuremberg, argued on the contrary that experiment wasn't a deviation foreign to standard practice but was inherent in it and required for it.

Ladimer and others tried a different tack to make experiment less legally perilous. The way the common law addressed peril required an update. Experiment, Ladimer argued, should be considered not a deviation from practice but a different kind of practice altogether. It was a structured, separate activity quite different from usual medical practice. He defined it as "a sequence resulting from an active determination to pursue a certain course and to record and interpret the ensuing observations."[100]

But attempts like Ladimer's to specify the differences between normal medical hypothesis testing and "experiment"—based on distinctive features such as institutional setting or the processes of patient recruitment— generally faltered. The therapeutic/nontherapeutic distinction instead persevered to structure how research was conducted. Even Ladimer vacillated between portrayals of research as a distinct practice, and research as a nontherapeutic part of medicine managed within broader norms of medical conduct.[101]

The randomized clinical trial was put forward as the new gold standard for medical research beginning in the 1940s and 1950s. A randomized trial was presumably a distinct practice. Research in this case was different in kind from clinical care. But during this period, early architects of these research trial designs nonetheless often continued to describe appropriate levels of scrutiny and consent required of research through therapeutic/nontherapeutic distinctions. An ethical trial was one that most closely resembled the real-world ambiguities inherent in making choices about treatment that physicians presumably had experience navigating. Deviation from such usual medical practices in the case of nontherapeutic research meant more scrupulous review, justification, and subject participation as well as opportunities for ease of exit.[102] By the late 1950s and early 1960s, experiment for the purpose of finding knowledge alone (nontherapeutic research) was, by wide consensus, subject to certain restrictions: informed consent, convincing relevance of study, competence of researcher, use of animal experimentation first if appropriate, and so forth. Such restrictions were contrasted to those applied to treatments for the patient's therapeutic benefit.[103]

By the mid-1960s, legal scholars felt confident that a consensus about the law had moved far enough away from the peril idea. But concern remained with respect to the general absence of statutory or judicial traditions explicitly endorsing human experimentation, which was still generally construed to mean nontherapeutic study. "The law relating to clinical investigation," reported a 1968 *JAMA* column, "is largely unsettled. There is little statutory regulation, and many of the important issues have not been decided by the courts."[104] Instead of suggesting research was some new practice, as Ladimer did, Beecher's friends Paul Freund and Curran concluded it still made sense to take the ubiquity view. Freund and Curran argued in the pages of the *New England Journal of Medicine* that the best way to understand the status of experimentation in the law was to judge it within the broader expectations of the ethical physician. "In my own writings and those of Marcus Plante, of Michigan Law School," wrote Curran, "the position is taken that 'informed consent' is *not* a clear concept so developed by the courts that it can now be followed with security by the medical profession in patient-treatment decisions...Even less, then, in clinical investigation."[105] The solution to a world without peril, opined Freund, is the "great traditional safeguard in the field of medical experimentation...the disciplined fidelity of the physician to his patient...First of all, do not do injury."[106]

Physician and scientist Louis Lasagna, an authority on research design and often a prominent critic of his profession and of improper research practices, mused, in typical fashion:

> One wonders how many of medicine's greatest advances might have been delayed or prevented by the rigid application of informed consent...if we are concerned with the problem of risk and danger rather than the abstract trampling of human rights, we will need to [focus] the principle of informed consent in a host of *other* medical situations...if we are to rely on informed consent rather than the good judgment of the trained physician, we shall have to reorganize completely the practice of medicine.[107]

Lasagna made the connection between practices and values, and between the scope of change needed in practices in order for such a change in values as described here to make sense. The conduct of research would, indeed, be "reorganized" dramatically during and after the 1970s. Research was increasingly defined as a distinct activity through bureaucratic, regulatory, and institutional requirements and routines specific to it. These made Ladimer's conditions of "difference-in-kind" not arguments, but realities. During the 1960s it was common to hear charges that Food and Drug Administration (FDA) requirements of consent undermined patient safety; that Nuremberg created an impossible ideal and did not address the lessons learned from the Nazi experience as to the potential claim of social interest on pressures to participate in needed research; and that National Institutes of Health and Public Health Service requirements for research review committees actually privileged investigator-driven, not subject-centered, criteria.[108] But each of these views gave way, in turn, to a normalization of Institutional Review Board (IRB) routines, to the dominance of informed consent in framing research ethics, to widening the scope of research open to IRB committee scrutiny, and to an assumption that FDA practices and randomized, placebo-controlled trials represented a scientific gold standard of practice after being highly contested as such in the preceding decades. Widespread *belief* that research (therapeutic or not) was a distinct enterprise not intrinsic to practice and with separate rules and procedures, first required the sorts of changes that indeed *made* research a distinct enterprise—for example, the intensive capitalization, bureaucratization, and technocratic management of medicine and medical knowledge. These developments, in turn, supported the broader distribution, sourcing, and standardization of medical knowledge in the decades following the 1960s.[109] Framing research ethics differently worked when the conditions of work and knowledge production changed.

Efforts, especially since the 1970s, to challenge paternalistic decision making and privileged judgment and to open up medical accountability are to be celebrated and strengthened. But my interest in these developments comes not from what they mean ethically but what they do substantively: how they can potentially make medical knowledge better in terms of the "styles of thought,"[110] categories of explanation, points of view, driving questions, and rules to verify evidence that comprise it. The close interaction seen in these prior decades, and in centuries before, between positions around how medical knowledge is created, and the values and expectations guiding the conduct of care, deserve our attention.[111] It suggests that re-engineering how medical inquiry knows things has to be part and parcel if not preliminary to any deeper change in the moral experience or accountability of care. Medical epistemology is wrapped up with moral position in the context of care.

In that respect I will argue that bioethics was actually *not bold enough* in driving needed innovation in how to generate and use medical knowledge. In the case of brain death, for example, a focus on bioethical tools of conceptual description and classification of brain states and meanings of personhood as a way to test the criteria, took on the surface but not the depth of the problems that ostensibly drove their advocacy and use. Uncertainty, ambivalence, and strangeness, persisted. Treating brain death as a problem of ethics analysis did not solve the kinds of challenges of managing medical work and knowledge for which older practices and values around omission, ordinariness, truthfulness, or therapeutic benefit were a response. Those practices remain a resource for curiosity rather than caricature, for a broader dialogue about how to do better in addressing what is hard about generating and using medical facts.

Before picking up these themes further later in this book, I first ask how Beecher took this background of prior medical decision making and experiment to arrive at brain death—how practice and value interrelated for him. Beecher relied on these familiar categories, but he took them on in new ways as well. He did so especially in response to how the brain-dead body erased familiar categories of medical explanation such that it not only compelled withdrawal of treatment but was no longer alive in that context.

NOTES

1. Robert Young, interview with the author, July 25, 1991; Ad Hoc Committee of the Harvard Medical School to Examine the Definition of Brain Death, "A definition of irreversible coma," *Journal of the American Medical Association* 205, no. 6 (August 5, 1968): 337–40.

2. Helmut Thielicke, "The doctor as judge of who shall live and who shall die," in *Who Shall Live; Medicine, Technology and Ethics*, ed. Kenneth Vaux (Philadelphia: Fortress Press, 1970): 146–94, 148.

3. Martin S. Pernick, "Back from the grave: recurring controversies over defining and diagnosing death in history," in *Death: Beyond Whole-Brain Criteria*, ed. Richard M. Zaner (Dordrecht: Kluwer Academic Publishers, 1988), 7–74, 60.

4. Vanessa Harding, "Whose body? A study of attitudes towards the dead body in early modern Paris," in *The Place of the Dead: Death and Remembrance in Late Medieval and Early Modern Europe*, eds. Bruce Gordon and Peter Marshall (Cambridge: Cambridge University Press, 2000), 170–87, 171.

5. Ad Hoc Committee, 337.

6. Beecher to Ebert, Box 6, Folder 17, Beecher Papers, The Harvard Medical Library in the Countway Library of medicine, Boston, MA.

7. Beecher to Folch-pi, Curran, Box 6, Folder 80, Beecher Papers.

8. Beecher to Curran, June 14, 1967 and June 23, 1967, Box 11, Folder 17, Beecher Papers.

9. Beecher to Curran, June 23, 1967, Box 11, Folder 17, Beecher Papers.

10. Beecher to Murray, Box 6, Folder 21, Beecher Papers.

11. Beecher to Ebert, October 30, 1967, Box 6, Folder 17, Beecher Papers.

12. Ebert to Beecher, November 3, 1967, Box 6, Folder 17, Beecher Papers.

13. Ebert memorandum, Box 6, Folder 17, Beecher Papers. Potter was actually appointed later as Beecher bemoaned to Ebert subsequently the unresolved lack of a theologian. See Beecher to Ebert, January 9, 1968, ibid.

14. Eelco F. M. Wijdiks, "The neurologist and Harvard criteria for brain death," *Neurology* 61 (2003): 970. See also Calixto Machado, *Brain Death–A Reappraisal* (New York: Springer, 2007).

15. Ebert to Beecher, Box 6, Folder 17, Beecher Papers.

16. Transplantation was not a central concern to the Committee. Briefly put: the fate of Curran's contribution to the Report, which began as an explicit response to the issues raised by transplant, was rejected by the Committee, as discussed in Chapter Three. MGH neurosurgeon Sweet failed, by his own account and supported by Committee archives, in his efforts as the only Committee member who purposefully sought to loosen the criteria explicitly in order to enhance transplant, as discussed in Chapter Five. The purposes, motives, and decades-long efforts and interests of Beecher and MGH neurologist Robert Schwab, who devised the essential elements of the criteria, show no indication of an interest in transplant but if anything do underscore an interest in setting limits to excessive uses of medical technology. Their work is discussed respectively later in the next chapter and in Chapters Four and Five. Other recollections and evidence support these interpretations as well.

It is striking to me how scholars who are familiar with Ebert's authorizing letter assume his words were aimed to smooth the path for transplantation. But the plain words simply do not convey that. Given the context that will unfold as summarized above, Ebert was arguably also more concerned about transplant and eager to see more responsible guidelines to police its use.

17. M. L. Tina Stevens, "Redefining death in America, 1968," *Caduceus*, Winter 1995, 207–19, 217. Also see Stevens, "The Quinlan case revisited: a history of the cultural politics of medicine and law," *Journal of Health Politics, Policy and Law* 21, no. 2 (Summer 1996): 347–66, and *Bioethics in America* (Baltimore, MD: Johns Hopkins University Press, 2000).

18. Albert Jonsen, *The Birth of Bioethics* (New York: Oxford University Press, 1998).

19. Peter Singer, *Rethinking Life and Death* (New York: St. Martin's Press, 1994), 25.

20. One of the most accomplished scholars of the culture and emergence of brain death repeats this position as well. Margaret Lock, *Twice Dead: Organ Transplants and the Reinvention of Death* (Berkeley: University of California Press, 2002). This view also formed the core of critiques of the Committee's work aimed at more general audiences. See Dick Teresi's typical *The Undead* (New York: Pantheon Press, 2012).

21. Exceptions include Wijdicks, "The neurologist and Harvard criteria for brain death." Most efforts to engage this detail, however, often misread it. The gradual consolidation of the Beecher archive itself, and limited availability of material from medical records and key actors such as Schwab, also contributes to this. Mita Giacomini, "A change of heart and a change of mind? Technology and the redefinition of death in 1968," *Social Science and Medicine* 44, no. 10 (1997): 1465–82. For example, Giacomini quotes—and then medical anthropologist Margaret Lock and others (Scott Henderson more recently, and discussed here in Chapter Six) have subsequently re-quoted—a section of a memorandum that Curran prepared for the Committee, which is the subject of Chapter Three. Curran argued that brain death would be inadequate to overcome possible legal obstacles to transplantation. Although the passage has been interpreted by these writers to demonstrate a transplant preoccupation, when put in context—of the Committee's rejection of the more expansive approach Curran suggested, recollections of Committee members, and other actions by the Committee and Beecher in drafting the document—the memo instead outlines a direction and a preoccupation that the Report *avoided* rather than embraced. Martin Pernick—eschewing the presentist tendency to critique the Committee when it is criticized as practical rather than conceptually pure—was able to see the Committee's interest in transplant as part of a broader view that linked judicious resource use and worthwhile innovation. Martin Pernick, "Brain death in a cultural context: the reconstruction of death, 1967–1981," in *The Definition of Death: Contemporary Controversies*, eds. S. J. Younger, et al. (Baltimore, MD: Johns Hopkins University Press, 1999), 3–33.

22. Box 6, Folder 23, Beecher Papers.

23. John Bunker, "Henry K. Beecher," in *The Genesis of Contemporary American Anesthesiology*, eds. Perry P. Volpitto and Leroy D. Vandam (Springfield, IL: Charles C. Thomas, 1982), 104–19.

24. Beecher remained active until his death in 1976. He wrote an authoritative history of Harvard Medical School, published and lectured on brain death, and completed, as will be detailed later in this study, a second book on human experimentation.

25. Curran to Beecher, October 27, 1958, Box 11, Folder 16, Beecher Papers.

26. MGH, Medical Records. Medical case records reviewed throughout this book will not be singularly referenced as to source other than noting the date and describing content, as part of maintaining confidentiality of identities and conforming to rules of use and MGH IRB approval for this purpose.

27. Schwab complemented his training in medicine at MGH with exposure to neuro-pathology at the University of Munich and psychiatry at the Boston Psychopathic Hospital, before returning to MGH in the mid-1930s. He died in 1972. See, John S. Barlow, Obituary, *Journal of the Neurological Sciences* 19 (1973): 257–58.

28. Robert Young, Obituary, "Robert S. Schwab, M.D. 1903–1972," *Archives of Neurology* 27 (September 1972): 271–72.

29. Ian Dowbiggin, *A Merciful End: The Euthanasia Movement in Modern America* (New York: Oxford University Press, 2002).

30. There was significant debate over the value of the respirator for these two generally different circumstances, with efficacy generally considered far greater in the latter case.

31. See Henning Pontoppidan, "The development of respiratory care and the Respiratory Intensive Care Unit (RICU): a written oral history," in *"This Is No Humbug!" Reminiscences of the Department of Anesthesiology at the Massachusetts General Hospital*, ed. Richard J. Kitzler (Boston: MGH), 151–77.

32. Jack Emerson, interviews with the author, July 22, 1992 and August 4, 1992.

33. James C. Wilson, *American Journal of Diseases of Children* 43, no. 6 (June 1932): 1433–54.

34. John Harley Warner, *The Therapeutic Perspective: Medical Practice, Knowledge, and Identity in America, 1820–1885* (Cambridge: Harvard University Press, 1986).

35. Joel Howell, *Technology in the Hospital: Transforming Patient Care in the Early Twentieth Century* (Baltimore, MD: Johns Hopkins University Press, 1995).

36. Martin Pernick, *A Calculus of Suffering: Pain, Professionalism, and Anesthesia in Nineteenth Century America* (New York: Columbia University Press, 1985).

37. Anonymous, "A way of dying," *The Atlantic Monthly* 199, no. 1 (January 1957): 53– 55.

38. Editorial, "Life-in-death," *The New England Journal of Medicine* 256, no. 16 (April 18, 1957): 760–61.

39. Ian Dowbiggin, ⊠*A Merciful End: The Euthanasia Movement in Modern America* (New York: Oxford University Press, 2002).

40. Perrin H. Long, "On the quantity and quality of life," *Resident Physician* 6, no. 4 (April 1960): 69–70.

41. Frank J. Ayd Jr., "The hopeless case: medical and moral considerations," *JAMA* 181, (no. 13 September 29, 1962): 1099–1102, 1102.

42. Ayd, p. 1099.

43. Gerald Kelly, "The duty of using artificial means of preserving life," *Theological Studies* 11 (1950): 203–20.

44. Examples of other frequently quoted considerations of this question that appeared soon before Beecher sought to establish the Committee include G. Biorck, "On the definition of death," *World Medical Journal* 14 (September–October 1967): 137–39; J. Voigt, "The Criteria of Death," 143–46; "When Are You Really Dead?," *Newsweek*, December 18, 1967; Arthur Winter, ed., *The Moment of Death* (Springfield, IL: Charles C. Thomas, 1967); Frank J. Ayd Jr., "When Is a Person Dead?," *Medical Science* 18, no. 33: 33–37.

45. William P. Williamson, "Life or death—whose decision?," *JAMA* 197, no. 10 (September 5, 1966): 139–41, 139.

46. Editor, "What and when is death," *JAMA* 204, no.6 (May 6, 1968): 539–40.

47. M. Martin Halley and William F. Harvey, "Medical vs. legal definitions of death," *JAMA* 204, no. 6 (May 6, 1968): 423–25, 423. A similar analysis was in M. Martin Halley and William F. Harvey, "On an interdisciplinary solution to the legal-medical definitional dilemma in death," *Indiana Legal Forum* 2 (1968–1969): 219–37.

48. Pope Pius XII, "The prolongation of life," *Pope Speaks*, November 24, 1957, 393–98, 397.

49. Halley and Harvey, "Medical vs. legal definitions of death," and "Law-medicine comment: definition of death," *Journal of Kansas Medicine Society* 69, no. 6 (June 1968): 280–82; "Law medicine comment: the definitional dilemma of death," *Journal of the Kansas Bar Association* 37 (Fall 1968): 179–85.

50. William F. Harvey, interview with the author, January 21, 2003.

51. Edward H. Rynearson, "You are standing at the bedside of a patient dying of untreatable cancer," *CA* 9 (June 1959): 85–87.

52. "Symposium on terminal care," *CA* (January-February 1960): 12–24, 20.

53. Alexander Brunschwing, "Radical resections of intra-abdominal cancer- summary of results in 100 patients," *Annals of Surgery* 122, no. 6 (December 1945): 923–32.

54. Meigs as an audience discussant of a paper by Whipple, in Allen O. Whipple, "Radical surgery in the treatment of cancer," *Annals of Surgery* 131, no.6 (June 1950): 812–23.

55. For a good summary and characterization of these individuals and perceptions of surgical therapeutic optimism, efficacy, and adventurism in this period, see Barron H. Lerner, *The Breast Cancer Wars: Hope, Fear, and the Pursuit of a Cure in Twentieth-Century America* (New York: Oxford University Press, 2001).

56. Harvey B. Stone, "The limitations of radical surgery in the treatment of cancer," *Surgery, Gynecology and Obstetrics* 92, no. 2, (August 1953): 129–34, 133, 134. See also his editorial "Limitations in the treatment of malignant diseases," 2–3.

57. Eugene G. Laforet, "The 'hopeless' case," *Archives of Internal Medicine* 112 (September 1963): 314–26, 318.

58. John C. Ford, J. E. Drew, "Advising radical surgery: a problem in medical morality," *JAMA* 151, no. 9 (February 28, 1953): 711–16.

59. Donald Oken, "What to tell cancer patients: a study of medical attitudes," *JAMA* 175, no. 13 (April 1, 1961): 1120–28; W. T. Fitts and I. S. Ravdin, "What Philadelphia physicians tell patients with cancer," *JAMA* (November 7, 1957); W. D. Kelly and S. R. Frieson, "Do cancer patients want to be told?," *Surgery* 27 (1950): 822; D. Rennick, "What should physicians tell cancer patients," *New Medical Materia* 2 (March 1960): 51–53, reported in Oken, supra.

60. Robert J. Samp and Anthony Curreri, "A questionnaire survey on public cancer education obtained from cancer patients and their families," *Cancer* 10 (March–April 1957): 382–84, and "How much to tell?," *Time* (November 3, 1961): 60. For similar findings of physicians' reluctance to tell and patients saying they mostly wanted to hear, almost a decade later, see Group for the Advancement of Psychiatry, *Death and Dying: Attitudes of Patient and Doctor*, vol. 5, symposium no. 11 (New York: 1965), 591–667.

61. Guy F. Robbins, Mary C. MacDonald, and George T. Pack, "Delay in the diagnosis and treatment of physicians with cancer," *Cancer* 6, no. 3 (May 1953): 624–26. See also Walter C. Alvarez, "How early do physicians diagnose cancer of the stomach in themselves? A study of the histories of 41 cases," *JAMA* 97, no. 2 (July 11, 1931): 77–83.

62. Nathan S. Kline and Julius Sobin, "The psychological management of cancer cases," *JAMA* 146, no. 17 (August 25, 1951): 1547–51, 1547–49.

63. H. Feifel, *The Meaning of Death* (New York: McGraw-Hill Book Company, Inc., 1959); Robert Fulton, *Death and Identity* (New York: John Wiley & Sons, Inc., 1965); B. G. Glaser and A. L. Strauss, *Awareness of Dying.* (Chicago: Aldine Publishing Company, 1966); and L. Pearson, ed., *Death and Dying* (Cleveland: The Press of Case Western Reserve University, 1969).

64. Harley C. Shands, Jacob Finesinger, Stanley Cobb, and Ruth Abrams, "Psychological mechanisms in patients with cancer," *Cancer* 4 (1951): 1159–70; Arthur M. Sutherland, Charles E. Orbach, Ruth B. Dyk, and Morton Bard, "I. The psychological impact of cancer and cancer surgery," *Cancer* 5 (1952): 857–72; Ruth D. Abrams and Jacob E. Finesinger, "Guilt reactions in patients with cancer," *Cancer* 6 (1953): 474–82; Arthur M. Sutherland and Charles E. Orbach, "Psychological impact of cancer and cancer surgery. II. Depressive reactions associated with surgery for cancer," *Cancer* 6 (1953): 958–62; Morton Bard and Arthur M. Sutherland, "Psychological impact of treatment of cancer and its treatment. VI. Adaptation to radical mastectomy," *Cancer* 8 (1955): 656–72; Marvin G. Drellich, Irving Bieber, and Arthur Sutherland, "The psychological impact of cancer and cancer surgery. VI. Adaptation to hysterectomy," *Cancer* 9 (1956): 1120–26; Arthur M. Sutherland, "Psychological impact of cancer and its therapy," *Medical Clinics of North America* 40 (1956): 705–20.

65. Arthur M. Sutherland, "Psychological impact of cancer and its therapy," 719–20.

66. An attempt reported in the American flagship journal *Cancer*, to see if they could devise a method by which psychiatrists could predict those patients who would manage full disclosure and those who would not. Bo Gerle, Gerde Lunden, and Philip Sandblom, "The patient with inoperable cancer from the psychiatric and social standpoints: a study of 101 patients," *Cancer* 13, no. 6 (November–December 1960): 1206–17.

67. William C. Alvarez, "Care of the dying," *JAMA* 150, no. 2 (September 13, 1952): 86–91.

68. John Trawick Jr., "The psychiatrist and the cancer patient," *Diseases of the Nervous System* (September 1950): 278–80, 280. "Why then," this author asked, "do we as physicians when faced with the 'dread condition' suddenly reverse our fields, drop

all the painstaking technical knowledge which we have so laboriously acquired and regress to a floundering, rejecting and improvised but dishonestly rationalized and sanctimoniously self-justified level of performance?," (p. 279). For another critique of the roots of awkward physician behavior with terminal patients and their own psychological needs, see Edward M. Litin, "Should the cancer patient be told?," *Postgraduate Medicine* 28, no. 5 (November 1960): 470–75. Here too is advice to generally tell, with disclosure and venting of fears openly seen as healthy and constructive goals. But again, this advice is balanced by other advice to weigh doing so in response to patients' needs and the expected impact of disclosure.

69. Paul Chodoff, "A psychiatric approach to the dying patient," *CA* (January–February 1960): 29–32, 31.

70. Bernard C. Meyer, "Should the patient know the truth?," *Journal of Mount Sinai Hospital New York* 20 (March–April 1954): 344–50, 349.

71. John Gregory, *Observations on the duties and offices of a physician; and on the method of prosecuting enquiries in philosophy.* (London: Printed for W. Strahan and T. Cadell, 1770).

72. Gary S. Belkin, "Moving beyond bioethics—history and the search for medical humanism," *Perspectives in Biology and Medicine* 47, no. 3 (Summer 2004): 372–85.

73. Gary S. Belkin, "History and bioethics: the uses of Thomas Percival," *Medical Humanities Review* 12, no. 2 (Fall 1998): 39–59. Many medical texts on truth-telling, whether strongly advocating or sharply criticizing withholding information, shared this characteristic of vetting their views within a set of questions characteristic as well of the mid-twentieth-century debates on truth-telling: How do physician actions and demeanor impact healing? Such illustrative texts include Northington Hooker, *Physician and Patient* (New York: Baker and Scribner, 1849); Richard C. Cabot, "The use of truth and falsehood in medicine: an experimental study," *American Medicine* 5 (1903): 344–49; and Joseph Collins, "Should doctors tell the truth?," *Harper's Monthly Magazine* 155, 1927, 320–26.

74. Samuel Standard and Helmuth Nathan, eds., *Should the Patient Know the Truth? A Response of Physicians, Clergymen, and Lawyers* (New York: Springer Publishing Co., Inc., 1955); "Symposium: what shall we tell the cancer patient?," *Proceedings of the Staff Meetings of the Mayo Clinic* 35, no. 10 (May 11, 1960): 239–57. James G. Wilders, "Should the cancer patient be told?," *JAMA* 200, no. 8 (May 22, 1967): 157; Bernard C. Meyer, "Truth and the physician," in *Ethical Issues in Medicine: The Role of the Physician in Today's Society*, ed. E. Fuller Torrey (Boston: Little, Brown, and Co., 1968), 161–77.

75. James T. Patterson, *The Dread Disease: Cancer and Modern American Culture* (Cambridge, MA: Harvard University Press, 1987); George Crile Jr., "A plea against blind fear of cancer," *Life* 30, October 31, 1955, 128–42.

76. Jay Katz, *The Silent World of Doctor and Patient* (New York: The Free Press, 1984).

77. *Salgo v. Leland Stanford, Jr. University Board of Trustees*, in 1957, and *Natanson vs. Kline* 350 P 2d 1093.

78. *Watson v. Clutts* 136 SE 2nd 617, 1964: 621.

79. *Hunt v. Bradshaw*, 242 NC 517, 1955: 521.

80. *Roberts v. Wood*, 206 F. Supp. 579: 583.

81. *Natanson v. Kline,* 1102.

82. Ibid., *Natanson,* 1103

83. Marcus L. Plante, "An analysis of 'informed consent,'" *Fordham Law Review* 36 (1968): 639–72.

84. Irving Ladimer and Roger W. Newman, eds., *Clinical Investigation in Medicine: Legal, Ethical and Moral Aspects* (Boston: Law-Medicine Research Institute, Boston University, 1963).

85. *Trials of War Criminals Before the Nuremberg Military Tribunals,* vol. 2 (Washington D.C.: U.S. Government Printing Office, 1950), 181–82.

86. For a more detailed review of the contributions of Ivy, Alexander, and their work in the context of discussions by physicians and others in the years leading up to the actual trials, see Paul J. Weindling, "The origins of informed consent: the International Scientific Commission on Medical War Crimes and the Nuremberg Code," *Bulletin of the History of Medicine* 75, no. 1 (Spring 2001): 37–71, and Weindling, *Nazi Medicine and the Nuremberg Trials: From Medical War Crimes to Informed Consent* (Basingstoke and New York: Palgrave Macmillan. 2004). See also Andrew C. Ivy, "Nazi war crimes of a medical nature," *Federation Bulletin* 33 (1947): 133–146, reprinted in *Ethics in Medicine: Historical Perspectives and Contemporary Concerns,* eds. Stanley Joel Reiser, Arthur J. Dyck, and William J. Curran (Cambridge, MA: MIT Press, 1977), 267–72.

87. Andrew C. Ivy, "Report from war crimes of a medical nature committed in Germany and elsewhere on German nationals of occupied countries by the Nazi regime during World War II," *AMA Archives,* quoted in Jonsen, *Birth of Bioethics,* 135.

88. A. C. Ivy, "The history and ethics of the use of human subjects in medical experiments," *Science* 108 (July 2, 1948): 1–5, 3.

89. Robert N. Proctor, "Nazi science and Nazi medical ethics: some myths and misconceptions," *Perspectives in Biology and Medicine* 43, no. 3 (Spring 2000): 335–46, 343, 344.

90. Robert A. Burt, *Death Is That Man Taking Names: Intersections of American Medicine, Law, and Culture* (Berkeley: University of California Press, 2002). See esp. 80–86.

91. See Susan Lederer, *Subjected to Science: Human Experimentation in America Before the Second World War* (Baltimore, MD: Johns Hopkins University Press, 1995).

92. Medical Research Council, "Responsibility in investigation on human subjects" (1963); World Medical Association, "Declaration of Helsinki" (1964); British Medical Association, "Experimental research on human beings" (1963); American Medical Association, "Ethical guidelines for clinical investigation" (1966), in *Encyclopedia of Bioethics,* vol. 4, ed. Warren T. Reich, "Appendix: Codes and Statements Related to Medical Ethics. Section II Directives for Human Experimentation" (New York: The Free Press, 1978), 1764–81.

93. "The voluntary consent of the human subject is absolutely essential. This means that the person involved should have the legal capacity to give consent; should be so situated as to be able to exercise free power of choice, without the intervention of any element of force, fraud, deceit, duress, overreaching, or other ulterior form of constraint or coercion; and should have sufficient knowledge and comprehension of the

elements of the subject matter involved as to enable him to make an understanding and enlightened decision. This latter element requires that before the acceptance of an affirmative decision by the experimental subject there should be made known to him the nature, duration and purpose of the experiment; the methods and means by which it is to be conducted; all inconveniences and hazards reasonably expected; and the effects upon his health or person which may possible come from his participation in the experiment." Quoted in Paul B. Beeson, Philip K. Bondy, Richard C. Donnelly, and John E. Smith, "Panel discussion: moral issues in clinical research," *Yale Journal of Biology and Medicine* 36 (June 1964): 455–76, 455.

94. See Samuel E. Stumpf, "Some moral dimensions of medicine," *Annals of Internal Medicine* 64, no. 2 (February 1966): 460–70, 468. I contest Stumpf's "first" status by Jonsen. An earlier paper is one on deception in experiments by James P. Scanlan. Here, Scanlan argued that any deception, i.e. incomplete informed consent, violated a Kantian respect for others. But if one turned to an alternative utilitarian teleology, any defense of deception fails because a utilitarian claim would balance a future benefit with a current harm. Since the benefit of the experiment is unknown (that is why there is an experiment), utilitarian claims are inappropriate for experimental ethics on their own terms. A likely rejoinder to this, in the context of writing on this issue, particularly by clinicians in the 1950s and 1960s, would be that (a) then all medical intervention with uncertain outcome is immoral; and (b) reasonably expected goals and purposes, especially in the face of very limited risk, permit a good enough utilitarian calculus. James P. Scanlan, "The Morality of Deception in Experiments," *Bucknell Review* 13, no. 1 (March 1965): 17–26. More important, however, is to point out how the "first" historical narrative employed by Jonsen uncritically privileges and defines bioethics as a unique, philosopher's, discourse. It ignores and fails to engage centuries, if not millennia, of philosophical and theological commentary on medicine.

95. Mindel C. Sheps, "Problems created in clinical evaluation of drug therapy," *Perspectives in Biology and Medicine* 5 (Spring 1962): 308–23. Typical of this sort of approach was a *JAMA* editorial that illustratively cited a study at Bellevue comparing postoperative infection incidence between patients who did, versus those who did not, receive antibiotics preoperatively. Since real practice faced no clear consensus about the safety of either approach, and use or non-use would not routinely be detailed by the surgeon to the patient, the experimental situation mimicked the real situation and thus no "superfluous" actions, like a uniquely prescribed or reviewed consent, were necessary. Maxwell Finland, "Ethics, consent and controlled clinical trial," *JAMA* 198, no. 6 (November 7, 1966): 637–38. Of note, this particular editorial was a critical response to a widely read and discussed criticism of inadequate use of informed consent by Beecher that appeared in the *New England Journal of Medicine* the same year, and which will be discussed more in the following chapter as part of seeing how Beecher both inherited but also revised a longstanding set of practices and justifications for ethical conduct.

96. John J. Lynch, "Symposium on the study of drugs in man. Part III. Human experimentation in medicine: moral aspects," *Clinical Pharmacology & Therapeutics* 1 (1960): 396–400, 396.

97. For example, prominent physician and future Chair of Medicine at Yale, Louis G. Welt, expressed the views of many when criticizing Rule 2 of the Code, which read: "The experiment should be such as to yield fruitful results for the good of society unprocurable by other methods or means of study...." Referring to Rule 2, Welt wrote, "this can be so readily translated into actions wherein the 'ends justify the means,' and to a frame of references wherein the inherent rights of the individual are jeopardized in the interests of the society or the state." See "Reflections on the problems of human experimentation," *Connecticut Medicine* 25, no. 2: 75–78, 76–77. See also Michael B. Shumkin, "The problem of human experimentation in human beings. I. The research worker's point of view," *Science* 117 (February 27, 1953): 205–7, for an often quoted critique of ever invoking society's interest in doing nontherapeutic research, but also how degrees of risk should correlate with degrees of protection.

98. See, for example, the argument by Donald Dietrich in "Legal implications of psychological research with human subjects," *Duke Law Journal* (1960): 265–74; William Bennet Bean, "A testament of duty: some strictures on moral responsibilities in clinical research," *Journal of Clinical and Laboratory Medicine* 39, no. 3 (1952): 3–9; Otto E. Guttentag, "The problem of experimentation on human beings – II. The physician's point of view," *Science* 117 (February 27, 1953): 207–10, 208.

99. Paul B. Beeson, et al, "Panel discussion: Moral issues in clinical research," 455, 457.

100. Michael B. Shimkin, "The problem of experimentation in human beings," *Science* 117 (February 27, 1953): 205–7, 205.

101. Irving Ladimer, "Ethical and legal aspects of medical research on human beings," *Journal of Public Health Law* 3 (1955): 467–511. See also Ladimer, "Human experimentation—medicolegal aspects," *New England Journal of Medicine* 257, no. 1 (July 4, 1957): 18–24.

102. For example, Austin Bradford Hill, "Medical ethics and controlled trials," *British Medical Journal* (April 20, 1963): 1043–49; T. F. Fox, "The ethics of clinical trials," *Medico-Legal Journal* 28 (1960): 132–41; Ladimer, "Ethical and legal aspects of medical research on human beings."

103. Burke W. Shartel and Marcus L. Plant, "Consent to experimental medical procedures: failure to follow standard procedures," Reprinted in. Irving Ladimer and Roger W. Newman, *Clinical Investigation in Medicine*, 223–30; Joseph Stetler and Robert R. Moritz, "Medical professional liability in general," chap. 19 in *Doctor, Patient and the Law*, 4th ed., eds. Ladimer and Newman (St. Louis: CV Mosby, 1962), 230–33; Richard P. Bergen, "Consent in clinical investigation," *JAMA* 203, no. 7 (February 12, 1968): 281–2, 281.

104. Richard P. Bergen, "Common law and clinical investigation," *JAMA* 203, no. 6 (February 5, 1968): 231–2.

105. William J. Curran, "The law and human experimentation," *New England Journal of Medicine* 275, no. 6 (August 11, 1966): 323–5, 324.

106. Paul Freund, "Problems in human experimentation," *New England Journal of Medicine* 273, no. 13 (September 23, 1965): 687–92, 689.

107. Louis Lasagna, *Life, Death and the Doctor* (New York: Alfred A. Knopf, 1968), 259, 261.
108. These views were held by, among others, Curran in "The law and human experimentation."
109. Gary S. Belkin, "Misconceived bioethics: the misconception of the therapeutic misconception," *International Journal of Psychiatry and the Law,* 29 (2006): 75–85.
110. Ludwig Fleck, *Genesis and Development of a Scientific Fact,* eds. Thaddeus J. Trenn and Robert K. Merton, trans. Fred Bradley and Thaddeus Trenn (Chicago: University of Chicago Press, [1935], 1979).
111. Gary S. Belkin, "Moving beyond bioethics."

2

The Justification: Beecher's Ethics

"There is an ambiguity, I say, about man's creativity. It was imposed upon him as a task of creation, yet involves at the same time a blasphemous denial of his creatureliness."

—HELMUT THIELICKE, *Theologian, 1969*

enry Beecher delivered the Fifth Bernard Eliasburg Memorial Lecture at Mount Sinai Hospital in New York City on December 6, 1967. His remarks, reported on the front page of *The New York Times,* were entitled "The Right to Be Let Alone; The Right to Die."[1] The subtitle, "Problems Created by the Hopelessly Unconscious Patient," indicates that this talk was an elaboration of his Human Subjects presentation barely a month earlier—the presentation that served as the springboard for the Ad Hoc Committee and reflected the thoughts likely on his mind when he wrote to Curran about "RIGHT(s)" the prior June. The presentation provided a map for the work of the Committee itself. Sections from it were repeated verbatim in early drafts of the Report and in an article Beecher published on this topic in the *New England Journal of Medicine* just weeks prior to publication of the Committee Report.[2]

Beecher opened by describing a visit he made to a hospital as a guest on rounds: "We were told about a man on their wards who had been hopelessly unconscious for more than a year. He got pneumonia. The question was, should he be treated? He was." Beecher disapproved, and he calculated the costs and bed days occupied by this patient without benefit:

> Remember, this man was hopelessly unconscious. Are we obliged to treat such an individual when he can be kept "alive" only by *extraordinary* means? Pope Pius XII answered that question plainly, clearly: "No, you are not," he said.[3]

Beecher's surviving Eliasburg manuscript drew clear connections between his decades of writing in human experimentation ethics and his interest in brain death. It included a first sketch of criteria, based on Schwab's research, which would also appear in the first full draft of the Report, dated April 11. The April 11 draft "Discussion" section, which laid out the justification for brain death, was taken almost entirely from the Eliasburg manuscript as well (Figure 2.1).

Returning to his visit on hospital rounds, Beecher noted that:

> It costs about $30,000 per year, probably more, to maintain such an individual. It is not, I insist, crass to speak of money in such a situation: Money *is* human life. If we had more money, we could save more lives. Remember, this man was hopelessly unconscious...Are we obliged to treat such an individual when he can be kept "alive" only by *extraordinary* means?...In the meantime...the consequences of treating this hopelessly unconscious man's pneumonia: If the average hospital stay is two weeks, then by occupying a bed for a year, such a patient has kept 26 others out of the hospital, others who are salvageable as this man is not. With the present critical shortage of hospital beds, the admission of patients, even those with cancer, may be delayed for some weeks...As medicine's power for prevention, for healing grows...it is evident that moral and ethical problems increase in kinds and in complexity. I think it may be profitable to take a look at the underlying situation. And to do this will require an examination of some underlying propositions.[3]

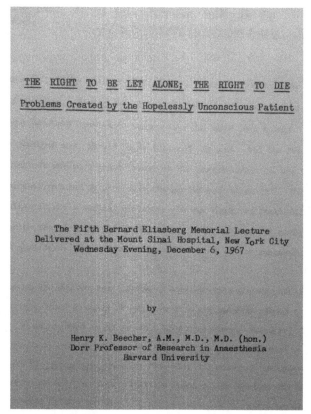

Figure 2.1 Eliasburg Manuscript Title Page Courtesy of The Harvard Medical Library in the Francis A. Countway Library of Medicine, Boston, MA.

For Beecher, who created the respiratory unit at Massachusetts General Hospital, these were real challenges. This early version of intensive care intensified the competing choices that new medical capabilities generated. The respirator salvaged life but also identified those who, because of medicine, become unsalvageable by medicine. The technology created an imperative to face up to its own consequences.

In the context of commonly held ideas about commission, therapeutics, and uncertainty—and especially in light of Beecher's experiences with experimentation ethics—a closer look at Beecher's "underlying propositions" can begin to address the question commonly launched at the Report: Why did seeming concern over the withdrawal of unnecessary treatment require a revised description of death? Beecher's first step was to consider threats from medicine to the idea of privacy, an idea he described as a unique accomplishment of the twentieth century. In his Eliasburg lecture, he quoted a paper by Edward A. Shils, titled "Social Inquiry and the Autonomy of the Individual,"[4] which warned of possible conflict between social science research on privacy and "self-determination…derived from our belief in the sacredness of individuality."[5] Beecher further observed a similar risk from all scientific study, arguing that "it is unthinkable to accept progress in medicine founded on deceit, on a subject defrauded of his privacy or his physical safety. Such runs counter to all that medicine stands for."[6]

In the paper Beecher quoted, Shils continued:

In this, the respect for human dignity and individuality shares an historical comradeship with the freedom of scientific inquiry, which is equally precious to modern liberalism. The tension between these values, so essential to each other in so many profoundly important ways, is one of the antinomies of modern liberalism.[7]

Shils also noted that autonomous individuality "is constituted by the feeling of being alive, consciously and continuously, by the existence of responsiveness which is part of a highly regulated system…This mindful, self-regulating core of the life of a human organism is what is sacred."[8]

So what was owed, what was "sacred" to the non-autonomous individual no longer in possession of conscious experience? It was in the context of these questions that Beecher then raised the issue of transplantation:

I mentioned Judge Cooley's memorable phrase (1888) that there is "the right to be let alone."…The individual's right to be let alone conflicts with the advancement of that part of society which is based upon scientific research…These thoughts and others to come are relevant to this presentation because of the pressures to use the hopelessly unconscious patient's tissues and organs in an attempt to help the otherwise hopelessly ill but still salvageable patient in certain experimental procedures…Certainly such individuals [in irreversible unconsciousness with no reflexes or response] have lost their ability to communicate. The question is, have they also lost their right to be let alone.[9]

In the Eliasburg lecture, the condition of hopeless coma and the tasks of setting limits on medical technology, autonomy, and transplantation are serially linked as problems of a similar type. These were problems of reconciling medical capabilities with obligations to persons, and Beecher addressed these problems using ideas gleaned over decades of experience in experimentation ethics practices. Experimentation provided a paradigm, a calculus, for balancing medical knowledge and medical power that could be applied to this new coma. Briefly put, for Beecher, brain death described a point at which medicine became unrecognizable experimentation.

BEECHER, EXPERIMENTATION, AND ETHICS

Beecher shared a longstanding approach to ethical conduct in medicine, summarized in the last chapter, that emphasized the contingent and hypothesis-testing nature of medicine and medical knowledge and the role of the physician as, in large part, an experimenter. In June 1965 Beecher, who chaired the MGH Subcommittee on Human Studies of its Committee on Research, was appointed by medical school dean George Packer Berry to what was then called the Ad Hoc Committee on Experimentation of Harvard Medical School, which was subsequently the Harvard Faculty Standing Committee on Human Studies. A few months later Beecher was named its chairman.[10] The fact that the ad hoc committee that described brain death was established as a subcommittee of Beecher's Harvard Faculty Standing Committee on Human Studies provides one of the more tangible connections between brain death criteria and rules about human experimentation. Beecher explicitly described the brain death Report as a product of the Human Studies Committee. In an update he prepared for the medical school faculty, Beecher highlighted that Report as the Human Studies Committee's most significant accomplishment.[11]

Beecher was internationally known for his interest in ethics and human experimentation. Through a series of writings, sandwiched between two books on the subject in 1958 and 1970, he offered ideas about the conduct of human experimentation that came out of his own clinical and research interest in anesthesia and the measurement of analgesic effects.[12] He wrote dozens of papers as well as a seminal book examining the mechanism and effectiveness of analgesia.[13] Scientific study of the effectiveness of analgesics required techniques that could measure subjective responses. One of Beecher's contributions was to develop those techniques. He was impressed with how the placebo effect could distort any effort to measure analgesic effects, especially if the object of study was, precisely, the phenomenon of suggestion itself. Alerting the subject to the purpose, potential use, and presence of placebo, especially when studying placebo, could get in the way of a reliable understanding of the real value of often dangerous treatments—for example, painkillers—against which placebo was compared:

> When a patient places himself in the hands of a physician for relief of a symptom or cure of a disease, this act implies consent to the physician to carry out all necessary means to relieve or cure. If the problem is pain...placebo will often relieve half to two-thirds of the pain relievable with an optimal dose of morphine. Surely, it would be carrying matters too far to require a dissertation to the patient on grades or degrees of relief anticipated, when real value could be expected from the use of a placebo.[14]

Beecher's research also suggested that in rating the severity of a painful stimulus, the response to analgesics differed depending upon whether the subjects were sick and in pain or whether they were healthy. He concluded that the analgesic potency of morphine, or of a placebo, depended upon context. The placebo effect was most powerful in the context of pain, disability, and fear:

> The greater effectiveness of the placebo where the stress and reaction are greatest, taking into account that the placebo can only act on the

reaction facet, supports the view that placebos being chiefly effective as indicated when there is great significance, great reaction, do indeed act by altering the reaction.[15]

If informed consent could contaminate the very object of investigation, as well as the mechanism of benefit and relief, then the right balance between consent and benefit was harder to pull off than it looked. The ideal of informed consent was just that, and in light of this data Beecher shared much of the skepticism of his contemporaries. Also in line with most of his contemporaries, Beecher emphasized the value of the therapeutic/ nontherapeutic distinction to guide physician conduct during research. When "experiment" more closely approached "routine" (therapeutic) care, acceptance by the patient of a physician's care meant consent:

> The central conclusion is that it is unethical and immoral to carry out potentially dangerous experiments without the subject's knowledge and permission. Every act of a physician designed soundly to relieve or cure a given patient is experimentation of an easily justifiable kind. The patient's placement of himself in the physician's hands is evidence of consent. The problem becomes a knotty one when the acts of the physician are not directed toward the benefit of the patient present but towards patients in general. Such action requires explicit consent of the patient.[16]

Reacting to the first rule of the Nuremberg Code that the subject "should have sufficient knowledge and comprehension of the elements of the subject matter involved so as to enable him to make an understanding and enlightened decision," Beecher wrote:

> Practically, this is often quite impossible...for the complexities of essential medical research have reached the point where the full implications and possible hazards cannot always be known to anyone and are often communicable only to a few informed investigators and sometimes not even to them.[17]

Over the next fifteen years Beecher continued to write and speak on experimentation ethics, culminating in his 1970 book *Research and the Individual*,[18] much of which was a patchwork of excerpts from papers published over that period.[19] In this work, he tended to describe a conditional commitment to informed consent. While informed consent was expected in all cases, especially as it "increased respect for the individual by providing him with opportunities for self-determination,"[20] nonetheless, "the patient who goes to a physician for relief consents, in the very act of going, to reasonable efforts to treat him...When a patient places himself in the hands of a physician for relief of a symptom...this act implies consent to the physician to carry out all necessary and acceptable means."[21]

Deliberations of the Human Studies Committee at Harvard show the regular use of these ideas under Beecher's leadership.[22] For example, a Human Studies Committee "Policy for informed consent in double-blind studies" dated July 21, 1966, concluded that if such studies, which were still controversial,[23] compared a generally accepted treatment against an unknown one, the study needed full informed consent subject to review by Human Studies Committee. If, however, there was no accepted treatment and the research involved testing an intervention against a placebo, the primary issue for human studies review was the adequacy with which the investigator understood and presented the ratio of risk to benefit. If there was no discernible risk, and a placebo might reasonably be expected to have equivalent value to the tested intervention, then, in ethical terms, testing this intervention was equivalent to using new but "unproven remedies in individual patients in a doctor–patient relationship. In such cases informed consent would be unnecessary and quite likely to distort the reactions of patients." Next to this sentence in the policy, Beecher added, in his own hand, "consent having been given in the coming of the patient to the physician."

The Human Studies Committee minutes contain the oft-repeated phrase "usual doctor–patient relationship," which provided the substantive branching point of a decision tree of ethical decision making and scrutiny. So, in one study simple blood tests might need consent, since taking blood for the particular purpose at hand was not a practice found in the "usual doctor–patient relationship." On the other hand, a study that used biopsy materials taken in the usual course of diagnosis of breast lesions, for example, did not need specific forms or review of informed consent. Informed consent was up to the physician. The central purpose of any medical ethic, as Beecher understood it, was to recognize when one was practicing as a physician for a patient's benefit and when one was not. The uncertainty and contingency of much of medical knowledge underscored this.

The debate decades later over clinical equipoise—the idea that the ethical design of a research trial hinged on whether it was offering options that held "equal position" in terms of knowing which course of treatment or intervention was preferred—indicates the longevity, rather than the anachronism, of the positions Beecher and his contemporaries took and of the problems they engaged.[24] That (ongoing) debate revisited the same themes reviewed in the prior chapter as to whether research and clinical responsibilities were indeed different in kind. It also underscored how faith in consent as a primary safeguard hinged on different understandings of the uncertainty of medical knowledge.[25]

Beecher's position—that judgment about disclosure and therapeutic equipoise inevitably rested with physicians, rather than being more broadly shared and determined—was common for the period.[26] But he joined this position with efforts to make professional practice more transparent. Beecher took public aim at colleagues for inadequate consent that failed to live up to the obligations of performing nontherapeutic research. He essentially accused leaders of a study of abnormal heart rhythms of flouting legal obligations to patients. The study's leaders, in contrast, argued that they had explained the procedure of inducing arrhythmias, but—since it was impossible to transmit the full background and depth of information necessary to assess the risks—that they had consequently "accepted the role of guarantor of the patient's rights and safety." Beecher argued that despite the understanding that fully informed consent is a "chimera…the fact remains that informed consent is a *goal toward which we must strive.*" The "adoption of the paternalistic view…leaves…what should be a joint enterprise between subject and investigator...a monopoly of the investigator."[27]

His critique broadened. Among his most famous papers is one which historian David Rothman considered a seminal event in the creation of bioethics. Titled "Ethics and Clinical Research," the paper detailed twenty-two studies (whittled down from fifty) chosen from the medical literature; each of the chosen studies had exhibited unacceptable breaches of informed consent and additionally had posed harm to patients. Beecher kept then Harvard Medical School Dean Berry informed of this sensitive work as it progressed: "As I delve deeper into this business the story is even more shocking than earlier seemed the case."[28] Drafts were shared with Berry, but Beecher took pains to later ask that Berry return the forwarded copies and identified specific people to whom he expressly asked that Berry make no mention of the work.

This approach to consent, involving great discretion by the therapeutic physician along with great censure to breaches of the obligation of consent, was grounded in the broader legal and medical thinking about human experimentation, which emphasized the overall experimental nature of medical knowledge and distinguished therapeutic from nontherapeutic interventions.

Beecher's public critiques and the use of large-outcome datasets reflected an interest in quality and accountability that were unusual for the time. The "exposé" in *The New England Journal of Medicine* was not Beecher's first stint as a critic of colleagues. He orchestrated a study published in 1954 of surgical mortality to determine the role of anesthesia practices in such deaths. This was a uniquely large, multicenter, collaborative effort for this period and was unusual as well in its specific intent to fix responsibility for poor outcomes on physicians and to capture such outcomes through the large-scale and public use of data. One of the more controversial findings was that significant mortality was due to the use of curare, and the report led to significant changes in practice. It also generated significant controversy, given the publicity surrounding it.[29]

Beecher's writings and comments about experimentation, along with the work of the Human Studies Committee itself, reveal a mix of significant caution and strong but poorly detailed affirmations of informed consent as a standard and fundamental practice. This ambiguity reflects less Beecher's lack of analysis than his focus on avoiding harm given the presumed larger perils and responsibilities of medical decision making. Fundamentally, the struggle over informed consent that Beecher shared with many of his contemporaries was driven by the experience that *harm* was a more significant issue than *consent*, especially when consent was not considered to be a reliable guarantor of the avoidance of harm. While consent was critical, it was not the foundational safeguard. Inevitable reliance on physician judgment—given the inevitable limits of patient expertise, especially in a context of knowledge that was frequently uncertain to begin with—required much of physicians in return. As Beecher wrote in a 1966 address, "Medicine without complete integrity can become a malignant craft."[30]

Beecher added to this background of consent and experiment, as well as a shared understanding of the contingency and responsibilities of managing medical facts, a particular synthesis of views about science and values. This substantially broadened his understanding of physician obligation and equipoise and provided a framework for addressing the issues raised in Eliasburg. In a closing chapter of *Research and the Individual*, Beecher brought together ideas (not emphasized in his prior writing on experimentation) on the relationship between science and ethics and on the distinction between treating patients as means or as ends. He cited Immanuel Kant, whose foundational work in moral philosophy of course placed means–ends distinctions at the core of moral action. He also briefly summarized controversy over naturalistic ethics; that is, the idea that science *is* ethics in the sense of realizing and revealing the natural relations between things for knowledge of right action.[31] Beecher did not subscribe fully to that view, nor a related Darwinian ethics in which the good was revealed through the surviving natural order. Instead, he described a relationship between ethics and science whereby science essentially framed ethical choices along a reasonable range of outcomes, harms, and tradeoffs that one might expect based on a given choice, such as the option to utilize a new medical technology.

"Harm" was not abstract. It was an unavoidably slippery term and needed empirical foundation. Harm was also accompanied by the inherent problem of position: Who was best positioned to describe and decide about relevant harms? In a section entitled "Statistical Morality" in the last pages of *Research and the Individual*, Beecher noted how any intervention, whether regarded as "routine" or "experimental," contained some danger and some benefit, which could only be compared in degree. "It has been calculated," he offered in one example, "that while the effects of [routine chest X-rays in Britain in 1957] might possibly have caused as many as 20 cases of leukemia in that year, nevertheless the examinations revealed 18,000 cases of pulmonary tuberculosis, as well as thousands of other abnormalities."[32] The actual numbers mattered. The specific tradeoffs, losses, and gains were relevant. This was especially true for a medical decision involving a calculus of therapeutic benefit. In the earlier pages of *Research and the Individual*, Beecher had counseled against forced experimentation with risk to one individual for knowledge to benefit one million; nonetheless, at the close of this book he approvingly recalled the decision made by Allied forces in North Africa during WWII to use precious stocks of the antibiotic streptomycin to treat soldiers with venereal disease rather than the seriously wounded. In this way, "salvageable" men could go back and fight. The situation mattered and, for Beecher, the role of science in ethics was as its starting point—to describe the situation. Without informed beneficence—known within the context of practice and supported through data—ethics was blind.

Beecher specifically endorsed the work of Joseph Fletcher, moral theologian and author of *Situation Ethics* and a number of other works that criticized the rule-oriented focus of much of Christian moral theology. Fletcher also wrote *Morals and Medicine*, often cited as a prelude to the modern bioethics movement. Beecher and Fletcher socialized often and engaged in a warm and casual correspondence. From the surviving archive, Fletcher appears to be the only person, other than Committee members and Ebert, with whom Beecher shared a copy of the Report prior to publication. The two also bonded over disagreements with theologian and philosopher Paul Ramsey, who would emerge as both a critic of brain death and an intellectual godfather to key figures in the nascent bioethics movement.[33]

Beecher gave Fletcher the credit for his own thinking about situational ethics: "Fletcher has thoroughly convinced me, who earlier thought to the contrary, that *only* the end justifies the means." Beecher reviewed Fletcher's use of G. E. Moore's 1903 *Principia Ethica* to argue that the terms such as "right" were only proxies for desired results. Given this argument, an action not justified by its results couldn't possibly be "right." If the *ends* did not justify the means, he asked, then what did? Yet Beecher's gloss on Fletcher contained an important clarification: "This is no place for a universal: not any end will justify any means...the means must be appropriate to the ends."[34]

Science could help mediate how to best judge the harms at stake—thus the reference to Kantian choice in Beecher's *Research and the Individual*. Choosing between what he described as Bertrand Russell's position—that ends are set by desire and science determines the means—and Kant's position—that people ought only be treated as ends in themselves—Beecher settled, through Fletcher, on an intermediate view. Quoting Jacob Bronowski, who portrayed science as not mere technique but as a method for collectively drawing conclusions about facts in a way that required creativity, tolerance, and respect, Beecher wrote that this is "the scientist's ethics, and the poet's and every creator's: that the end for which we work exists and is judged only by the means which we use to reach it."[35] However, at the same time, the specific ends at stake were critical. Means had to live up to their ends. Beecher's interest in desired results and ends was quite different than a Utilitarian maximization of the good. He demonstrated a more a nuanced understanding borne from his own clinical experience that the value of some results over others came from their fit with yet other results and values. Care and clarity in how results and means were described and the reliability of underlying knowledge tools to capture them, was essential. For Beecher, medical knowledge filled this role, and had to live up to it.

This principled pragmatism, informed by a naturalistic viewpoint, proves particularly interesting and potentially valuable in the context of later criticism of brain death and uses of bioethics in the following decades, reviewed in Chapter 6. Beecher's joining together of issues of futility, scarce resources, autonomy, transplant, and brain death in Eliasburg also made sense within this framework. Use of intrusive interventions to support a hopelessly unconscious patient without brain function was not justifiable as a means, *except* as an attempt to harvest organs for others. Beecher seemed more interested in determining what conditions in which life support was a justifiable means, than in promoting transplantation. Transplantation, which Beecher described as experimentation,[36] is best understood not as his driving goal but as the only end that could redeem the otherwise unjustifiably experimental continuation of life support in those patients. Otherwise, the boundaries and logic of medical knowledge creation and use were violated and no longer justifiable means.

CRITICS

Others read Beecher, and the whole project of evaluating brain death and appropriate medical intervention, quite differently. In a December 1970 forum on brain death sponsored by the American Academy for the Advancement of Science (AAAS), Beecher acknowledged that defining death as death of the brain was an "arbitrary" choice, in words that would be a magnet for future criticism:

> At whatever level we *choose* to call death, it is an arbitrary decision. Death of the heart. The hair still grows. Death of the brain? The heart may still beat. The need is to choose an irreversible state where the brain no longer functions. It is best to choose a level where, although the brain is dead, usefulness of other organs is still present.[37]

Any set of criteria was a choice. If forced to choose, he argued in his post-Fletcher mode, some choices lived up to their ends better than others.

The AAAS forum captured works in progress from members of a task force study group on defining death, convened by the newly organized

Institute of Society, Ethics and the Life Sciences, of which Beecher was an early member. The Institute, later named the Hastings Center, was founded by *Commonweal* editor Daniel Callahan and Columbia University psychiatrist Willard Gaylin in 1969, and was the first bioethics think tank. Robert Veatch, fresh from completing his doctorate, became its first employee and would later direct the soon-to-be-created Kennedy Institute of Ethics, itself founded in 1971. Veatch was arguably the earliest and most pointed critic of brain death and of the Committee in the years after the Report appeared; he considered the Committee's attempt to formulate any justification for brain death to be essentially irrelevant. It was not their role:

> The task of defining death is not a trivial exercise in coining the meaning of the term. Rather, it is an attempt to reach an understanding of the philosophical nature of man...to leave such decision-making in the hands of scientifically trained professionals is a dangerous move.[38]

Veatch targeted Beecher's acknowledgment of arbitrariness as either "capricious whim or crass expediency," and argued that determining an essential value or meaningful aspect of the human body, which we could then identify as lost in death, was "a matter where neither technical data nor personal preferences are relevant as evidence. We are dealing with a third category...the theological, the metaphysical...the ethical."[39]

Veatch's primary objection to brain death was that death was inappropriately understood as a clinical state or scientific fact. Instead, he argued, it was a question of meaning. What does the transition to death *mean*? To say someone has died can mean many different things—that someone no longer respires, reasons, socially interacts, integrates homeostatic mechanisms, has consciousness or flow of bodily fluid, etc. Veatch portrayed Beecher as taking the position that death meant loss of consciousness and, further, that Beecher had not adequately argued for privileging that meaning. The criteria were not valid simply because doctors declared it. Veatch suggested that given the range of meanings possible, public policy ought to permit individuals to specify which meaning they wanted applied to them. Brain death should not be used in cases where an individual had previously specified that this was not how they wanted their death defined, or for those who left no instructions.[40]

Veatch understood death as a "socio-ethical" fact that was mistakenly left in the hands of medical-technical experts. When physicians made distinctions about when death occurred, they only demonstrated the intrusion of their socio-ethical biases:

> Questions of what is valuable cannot be settled by an appeal to technical biological or medical evidence. We who are professionals are in danger of what I call the generalization of expertise when they make this error. Generalization of expertise is the attributing of special knowledge in all aspects of a problem area, including the ethical and philosophical aspects, to the person who has technical expertise in that area.[41]

In *Research and the Individual*, Beecher rejected a sharp separation between technical expertise and moral expertise about that technical expertise. The socio-ethical valence of medical facts might not be so readily expunged by trying to divide the labor of explanation amongst these different kinds of experts. The relationship between ends and means he arrived at with Fletcher made that separation incoherent but it also ironically acknowledged, in tandem with Veatch's stance, that medical facts—and in particular brain death—were sociocultural facts.

Much of the ethical and humanistic critiques of medicine in the following decades repeated this pattern: an assertion by critics of the situatedness or constructedness of meaning in practice, yet the desire to nonetheless create an objective, authoritative ethical or critical position and expertise over those meanings. Having one's objectivist authority cake, while eating a socio-relativist position too, can be tricky and would prove hard for bioethics to digest. That indigestion, seen in the later trajectory of the bioethical critique of brain death described in Chapter Six, draws attention to other solutions to manage complex medical facts, and thus potential alternative historical trajectories, from which to learn. Beecher and Schwab viewed the moral import of these facts as unavoidably part of their contingent nature, such that internal expertise and deep experience in their clinical context was a critical source of value and understanding.

Other early critics focused on the transplantation issue. Paul Ramsey's *Patient as Person* has often been considered with Fletcher's *Medicine and Morals* as a seminal work of modern bioethics, in that they both argued for patient autonomy. Ramsey lent his voice, as well, in the AAAS meeting and Institute Task Force. There, he primarily argued that the purpose of brain death criteria—to promote organ transplantation—was not moral, either in method or result.

At a different, earlier AAAS meeting on human experimentation, philosopher Hans Jonas presented a paper in response to Beecher's statement that society could ill afford to discard needed organs. Jonas' rejoinder was later recalled as one of the opening shots of the new presence of the philosopher in medicine, and as the establishment of a philosophical footing for the discussion of experimentation ethics.[42] Jonas disputed any interest on the part of "society":

> "Discarding" implies proprietary rights—nobody can discard what does not belong to him in the first place. Does society then own my body? "Salvaging" implies the same and, moreover, a use-value to the owner. Is the life-extension of certain individuals then a public interest?[43]

Jonas felt it was not. He criticized common justifications put forward for new medical technologies, because these justifications overshadowed the dignity and autonomy of individuals—and their ability to generate personal or particular values—by invoking the social benefits of these presumed advances. Jonas argued that "the destination of research is essentially melioristic. It does not serve preservation of the existing good from which I profit myself and to which I am obligated."[44] The capability to reduce harm and expand benefit for some did not, for Jonas, come with authority to make claims on others:

> What is it that *society* can or cannot afford...It surely can afford to lose numbers through death, it is built on the balance of death and birth decreed by the order of life...Society, in a subtler sense, cannot "afford" a single miscarriage of justice.[45]

Beecher agreed with this. But, as he argued directly here and in other forums, echoing earlier medical literature, Jonas then left no clear path as to how to progress—how to make new choices and seek innovation. The old problem of how medicine could or should continuously improve—a problem that drove appeals to values such as ordinariness, omission, therapeutic ends, and dispute over the purposes of consent—remained.

These exchanges captured core claims of the bioethics movement that followed. First among these was the claim that a wide array of philosophical and moral meanings were inappropriately assigned to medical categories, purposes, and areas of expertise. Death, according to this framework, was not a clear physiological process but a moral category made coherent by philosophy. Second, and relatedly, was a privileging of individual autonomy and choice in defining the ends and purposes of medicine. Diagnosis of brain death was a problem of misplaced expertise, and transplantation potentially sacrificed personal liberty for medical gain or discretion. Brain death, therefore, risked the individual in favor of society's medically driven search for progress.

Of course, lots of autonomous individuals would opt for lifesaving transplantation, and other progress. Beecher responded directly to Jonas, and both in print and in the marginalia of his copies of Ramsey's and Veatch's papers from the AAAS brain death panel. Beecher saw Jonas as "rationalizing people into the grave":

> The definition of brain death is not difficult. Isn't there something ominous, sinister, about a philosophy, a theology, that unquestionably exacts lives for the sake of an ill-defined philosophical principle?.[46]

Given the concerns he expressed in Eliasburg, and his views regarding the dangers of societal interests in experimentation ethics, Beecher likely felt that he needed no lecture from Jonas on the subject. When discussing Jonas's views, he would repeat his own shared aversion for posing society's betterment as a justification for medical research or treatment.[47]

Beecher also responded to the accusation that the definition of brain death was either morally presumptuous or morally bankrupt because of its connection to transplant. "The new definition will lead to saving countless lives. Isn't that 'morally' desirable? Denial will lead to death," he wrote in the margins of Ramsey's paper, which criticized the moral flaws of brain death's definition due to its supposed agenda of furthering transplantation.[48] Beecher was careful to underscore that these benefits, and any enhanced use of transplant, were "merely a *consequence* of the new definition."[49] He also held to his position that, irrespective of transplant, the moral consequences of brain death extended more broadly, arguing that "if beds are not cleared of corpses, cancer patients will be denied hospital admission."[50] For Beecher, these were moral consequences of brain death, not moral arguments for it.

But Beecher didn't directly answer Jonas' challenge as to the presumed value and inevitability of progress itself—a powerful challenge to the conduct of medical practice and the rationale for physician beneficence, but one that eventually faded as a focus of bioethics. The role of "calculator of suffering" ostensibly cast the physician as a gatekeeper who determined what types of progress could be considered worthy. Beecher and colleagues, as we have seen, did wrestle with this predicament—but Jonas and others argued to re-describe it altogether, to shift this predicament from doctor to patient. It was no longer *their* predicament as doctors: it was *ours*, as patients.

Wrestling over how to manage progress in medicine became less central to brain death debates, and arguably to bioethics. This mirrored a larger failure of consensus over the right tools for the management of medical progress on a broader scale, as evident in the acceleration of per capita costs in the US health care system relative to other systems, along with the decline in relative health gains that occurred in the United States in subsequent decades. Beecher's uses of standardization and pragmatism appear as responses precisely to this challenge of how to link medical knowledge with credible progress, and has affinities with other approaches that emerged in the latter twentieth and early twenty-first centuries to define health care quality and effectiveness. Notable among these are efforts that emerged in the 1980s to apply quality-improvement methods developed in the industrial sector to the field of health care (discussed further in Chapter Six). Along with other attempts to find science-driven strategies to manage medical facts (and in doing so to address social values and choice), these kinds of developments are important to discern and draw upon as a potentially distinct historical narrative of sourcing solutions to manage the progress and improvement of medicine through restructuring how knowledge is used by medicine. That framing narrative may prove more valuable for exploring strategies to manage the value-dimensions of medicine than the bioethics narrative has, as will be argued further in this book.

Beecher and Jonas actually had much to say to each other in a dialogue about social value, medical knowledge, and ambivalence about technological progress. Their specific conversation was short-lived, as was the limited degree to which their sort of exchange of ideas later drove bioethics in general and its approach to brain death in particular. Instead, the focus of the following decades of the brain death critique would lie not in what Daniel Callahan described as cultural questions about the trajectory of our technological society, but in questions about the nature of individual decisionmaking, autonomy, choice, and their conceptual features.[51]

In the decades following Beecher's career, vying concepts of death and personhood indeed became the focus of debate, falling within a range of views that could be located somewhere between Ramsey's position—that nature held moral constraints that could not be breached—and Veatch's position that describing nature's limits was often an excuse for acceding to medicine's subjective values.

More specifically, Ramsey questioned whether the Committee's argument for the acceptance of brain death rested on the natural death of the organism ("biological" death), the cessation of consciousness or, as Schwab concluded, both. Beecher cited Black's Law Dictionary definition, according to which "death occurs precisely when life ceases and does not occur until the heart stops beating and respiration ends. Death is not a continuous event and is an event that takes place at a precise time." He then considered a contrasting possibility:

> ...whether one believes that the individual's personality, his conscious life, his uniqueness, his capacity for remembering, judging, reasoning, acting, enjoying, worrying, and so on, reside in the brain, and that when the brain no longer functions the individual is dead. We have proof that these and other functions reside in the brain...It seems clear that when the brain no longer functions, when it is destroyed, so also is the individual destroyed; he no longer exists as a person: he is dead.[52]

Over fifteen years later, Veatch quoted these lines in order to underscore the point that Beecher and the Report really championed the conceptual position that loss of certain cognitive functions meant the death of the person but incorrectly presented that ethical or philosophical point of view as a medical fact.[53] Beecher instead had a more subtle view, understanding that the truth of brain death did not rest simply on either end of this conceptual spectrum. Schwab's development of the criteria, explored in subsequent chapters, also took place outside of this simple equation of unconsciousness, loss of personhood, and death. The Report itself defines "brain death," but also describes a kind of coma that involved much more than irreversible loss of remembering, judging, reasoning, or acting. In his comments to Beecher at AAAS, Veatch wrote: "I believe that Dr. Beecher sees the *meaning* of death as the loss of consciousness." On his copy of Veach's paper, Beecher responded, "no, loss of consciousness is the *result* of death." Schwab's experience applying brain death criteria to comatose patients with the use of EEG (also explored in following chapters), and his familiarity with a substantial body of EEG-based research on consciousness through the mid-twentieth century, reinforce the empirical incoherence with which Veatch's conceptual claims appear to have struck Beecher. In his remarks, Veatch argued that identifying the meaning of death requires deciding whether it is a process or an event; next to this passage, Beecher responded: "Both."[54] Veatch also described Beecher as having opted for consciousness as the significant value in defining life. Here, Beecher circled the word "significant" and wrote next to it "the ability to function." At the bottom of the page, he added: "How separate a functioning brain from the functions it performs?"[55] In his comments, irreversible loss of consciousness was considered the result of death, not the cause of it (irreversible loss of consciousness could occur in a non–brain dead patient). Consciousness, here, is a necessary but not sufficient property that must be lost for death to occur. But, as captured in Beecher's reference to brain functioning, consciousness is also one of several signals of the status of the brain, a neurologic symptom that Beecher accuses Veatch of failing to understand in his *conceptual* treatment of loss of consciousness. And where Veatch, in his AAAS response, referred to the lack of attention given to the meaning of death, Beecher wrote, "meaning and consequence are, I think, inseparable in a pragmatic society: 'things are what their results are.' "[56] Further on he added: "one would never dare turn off resp. of a living patient."[57]

In his report to the medical school faculty regarding the Ad Hoc Committee work as a product of the Human Studies Committee—perhaps reflecting what he saw as an emerging cognitive dissonance over the significance and use of the fact of irreversible loss of consciousness—Beecher noted, "I believed we were perhaps too timorous in calling our effort 'A Definition of Irreversible Coma' and not calling it brain death. I think we now should stress the fact that death of the brain is death indeed, even though the heart continues to beat."[58] But rather than titling the Report "brain death", it is Beecher's simple answer—"Both"—that more specifically reflects the concrete problem created by the conditions of death before dying, in which the physiologies of cardiopulmonary and brain function were separated and suspended so as to be able to fail in reverse order. This new kind of permanent loss of consciousness was a complex fact that included the neurologic state of a nonfunctioning brain—a necessary but not sufficient condition for the death of persons—as well as cardiopulmonary functions that were removed from any context of coherent medical action or survivability.

An important debate over medical knowledge was percolating here. Whatever the moral valences or conceptual creativity it inspired, this new body had to be managed in its functional concreteness. Through comments on manuscript marginalia, conference proceedings, and published papers, Beecher directly challenged Veatch's portrayal of the kinds of expertise and experiences required to define death. Alongside Veatch's description and indictment of medicine's faulty "generalization of expertise," we read Beecher's handwritten reply that "the philosopher and theologian have entered biology and make revealing statements. I would *never, never* reverse the process!"[59] Where Veatch criticized medical experts for deciding social policies, Beecher wrote: "Is the philosopher or theologian better equipped for this role?"[60] Elsewhere, Beecher noted that "these arguments, statements, etc. reveal how irrelevant 'philosophy' of this kind is to intellectual life."[61]

These manuscripts, letters, and papers further underscore the pragmatism or, as Beecher put it, the weighing of ends and means derived from situational ethics, which he ascribed to his friend Fletcher:

> In this world there are a number of imponderables most the least of which is situation ethics, so eloquently described by Professor Joseph Fletcher...If I may be permitted an over-simplification, it is a world where circumstances alter cases, a pragmatic world where things are what their results are. I realize I can easily get myself into hot water with the philosophers.[62]

This approach fit well with his work on experimentation and his understanding of the realities of choice and calculus at the root of all medical decision making. By working from within the choices and testable circumstances at stake, the criteria captured both the adequate necessity of unconsciousness *and* the adequate sufficiency of biological disintegration; further, the criteria reflected how when these conditions, occurring together, were not recognized as death, *the continuation of support was no longer recognizable as medicine.* Veatch felt that if defining death indeed involved choices, the task instead required unique expertise in clarifying conceptual meanings and was not the business of physicians. For Beecher the fact of choice was ines-capable, a reflection of how death was biologically imprecise—a truth that held even in the heart-lung criteria and in most medical knowledge. The respirator-bound patient created conditions whereby a brain that could no longer function was dead; describing that point did not and could not rely on metaphysical conclusions or conceptual analysis. Nonsurvivability and permanent unconsciousness as markers of death were not concepts to be argued but experiences and practices grounded as coherent accounts within medical practice, experimentation, and use.

Beecher was clearer in these post-Report debates, more so than in the Report itself, that the irreversible coma described in the criteria was a description of death, not of futility that permitted removing care. While critics like Ramsey and Veatch were focused on describing the contours of acceptable withdrawal, Beecher insisted in marginal notes to their written comments that such elaboration was fine but not his point. Responding to Ramsey who wrote asking why the "terminal patient" lost a claim to medi-cal attention, Beecher circled "terminal patient" and wrote: "Confusion, confusion! The terminal patient is not dead…Thus the new definition merely clears [unreadable] and supports this necessary act."[63]

VEATCH'S PROJECT

Beecher and Veatch, along with other early critics of brain death, were arguing as much about fundamentally different views of ethics as they were about brain death. Veatch's concern about the "generalization of expertise" formed the core of his doctoral dissertation at Harvard, which he had only recently completed when he debated with Beecher at AAAS. Later published as *Value Freedom in Science and Technology*, Veatch's work combined two prominent streams of thought at the time: a medical sociology derived from the thinking of Talcott Parsons, which focused on revealing the structured roles at work in medical encounters, and the enthusiasm among moral philosophers for establishing the objectivity of ethical reasoning.

Veatch detailed how when doctors and patients met, each made decisions or interpreted information based on various factors that he diagrammed with boxes and lines to portray a "Medical Action System." Physician and patient were illustrated within their "organic," "psychological," "social," and "cultural" contexts, each with another link to either a profession or other subculture (e.g., family). Each of those links was, in turn, similarly embedded in further boxed categories. Doctor and patient resided in these variously constructed and variously connected roles and boxes when they met. They would evaluate a given decision, such as whether to use an oral contraceptive pill (OCP), differently and with different filters and "lines" of accountability and reference. Veatch's point with these diagrams was that there existed a sociological, analytical approach to the interaction of doctor and patient, explaining how their decisions were predicated on their respective diagrammed social roles and connections as illustrated by the boxes they were in or to which they were linked. This relativization of medical judgments and decisions was at the same time an objectification—Veatch literally diagrammed the socially framed workings of medical thought and action.

One of the goals of this work was to contribute to debunking what Veatch described as an enduring and mistaken tendency to elevate fact over value. Veatch traced the lineage of that tendency from Descartes through Locke and Newton, and then on to G. E. Moore, who refuted John Stuart Mill's belief that the "good" could be defined through empirical study of what is desired. That long tradition stripped the "ethical" of any real, factual status. Veatch argued instead for an objective discourse about ethics. One only needed to clarify the boxes.

Veatch referred in particular to the work of Roderick Firth and William Frankena. Firth's 1952 paper "Ethical Absolutism and the Ideal Observer" was used by Veatch, as it had been used by others, to argue that the "ethical" was an objective category of knowledge in that it had properties that compelled a feeling of requiredness, and thus a sort of factualness independent of the preferences of a given observer.[64] Firth specifically wanted to reclaim from skeptics Moore's famous contrast between describing something as yellow, as opposed to describing it as "good." To say something was "yellow," Moore observed, described a property of a yellow thing. Yellow in that sense was a proxy for our perception of a natural phenomenon of "light vibrations." "Good" could also be a property of things, but any effort to identify other naturally founded characteristics of "good" was really just an elaborated listing of interpreted feelings about "good." This was because, unlike yellow, good had no referent in a natural or mechanical process. To equate the perception of yellow with its reality was accurate; equating good's reality with the perception of it was not. The latter inference confused *agreement* about what counted as good with its factualness and led to what for Moore was a key error: a naturalistic fallacy.[65]

Firth argued that while this insight led away from a naturalistic ethics, it moved toward describing a more robust nonnaturalistic one—a stance that went farther, perhaps, than Moore himself was willing to go. To see yellow was to make a relational statement of the following type: to say a thing is yellow is to say something about how it would appear to a certain person under such-and-such circumstances. Ethics was no different. Veatch similarly drew on Frankena in building an analytical foundation for defining the good, post-Moore. Frankena and Veatch (and Firth) were objecting to a strong vein of skepticism in philosophy up to the mid-twentieth century, especially captured through writings such as those of A. J. Ayers and the emotivist and logical positivist schools. That tradition saw normative debates about ethics—the right, good, just, etcetera—as meaning nothing more than the preferred, enjoyed, liked, or despised. In *Ethics*, Frankena argued that if intuitions, emotions, or moral sentiments were indeed the underlying source of ethical commitments, then the experience of obligation that was considered a transparent part of ethical statements would neither be needed nor actively sought. Moral discourse instead strove to universalize beliefs through principled, non-egoistical discussion.[66] Veatch joined this effort to reclaim an objective position for ethical reasoning in order to sketch a method for describing the good that could be both impersonal and objective. Such work relied upon texts such as Firth's and Frankena's, whose philosophical trajectory could be said to have culminated in John Rawls' *Theory of Justice* in 1972.[67]

Doctors exerted expertise over what, to Veatch, were ethical and not medical questions, which required a different expertise. In making ethical statements, doctors appropriated forms of symbolization different from those used in medical works stating facts about the body, and thus strayed out of the range of their expertise. To ignore these boundaries, to not keep symbols in their rightful boxes with their rightful owners, was to commit Frankena's error of calling one thing by another category—what he called the "fallacy of the generalization of expertise." Medical ethics needed to be rescued from a professional expertise that had overreached its set of sanctioned tools.[68]

Veatch's critique of Beecher's brain death criteria as falsely ascribing a fact to a value therefore reflected a larger project. The Report was perfect material with which to show off the possibilities of a commitment to objective philosophy that could reconfigure the work of medicine along social roles and actions. Veatch was not only taking on Beecher, but seeking to further a particular mid-twentieth-century movement in moral philosophy as he embarked on his career.

Veatch was a Harvard Divinity School graduate and had completed a PhD in Religion and Society from Harvard. The Kennedy Center was led by moral theologians. Jonas's work started with interpreting the Christian Gnostic tradition. Dan Callahan was a Catholic intellectual who served as editor of Commonweal, the prominent lay Catholic intellectual and policy journal, before taking on the Hastings Center. Jonas and Callahan, along with other early framers of American bioethics, sought to extend the relevance of moral theology in an increasingly secularized world. If theology was to remain relevant, religious thought needed to incorporate other disciplines such as moral philosophy and sociology.

Callahan wrote at length about the Church and its internal struggles over participation in a seemingly more politically divisive, pluralistic, and secularized society.[69] His detailed study of abortion, which appeared in 1970, began with the voice of a troubled Catholic but quickly moved on to describe how the issue could and should be engaged through pluralistic value systems. The key, he argued, was a technique of moral investigation that methodically examined these value systems in order to arrive at

overlapping principles—or at least to clarify differences in order to facilitate a more shared and inclusive discussion and, hopefully, consensus.[70]

Soon after Beecher and his Committee completed their work, Callahan
spoke at one of a series of conferences that formed the 1969 volume,
Updating Life and Death. In that book he detailed a method of moral philosophy, apparent in *Abortion*, with which to approach profound questions such as what made life sacred. He described a process of collective
deliberation that started with identifying broad shared first-principles that
could be a foundation for consensus or at least maximize areas of common
ground as more specific applications of these principles were explored.
The role of ethical analysis was to first identify such widely-shared
first-order principles, such as the sacredness of life. These principles took
as their starting point shared consensus over basic issues that might apply
to many situations or controversies. From these, argued Callahan, should
flow rules that could be subsequently evaluated and justified to the degree
that they answered more specific controversies, but in a way that served or
enhanced the larger principle(s). These subsequent rules and subrules, and
the debate about their fidelity to the larger principle(s), required regular
reexamination as new rules proliferated and new circumstances appeared.
Callahan envisioned a deliberative process, expanding from these core
shared principles, in order to reach moral conclusions that would cut
across seemingly distinct issues and controversies. Such a process would
ostensibly identify a coherent approach to related issues such as population control, death defining, and birth control.[71] This process was needed
since a "religious foundation for normative principles...[was] no longer
tenable."[72]

Veatch also began seeking theological answers for social problems but
turned quickly to more secular solutions. His *Value Freedom* explored
controversy over the use of oral contraceptives in great detail. He studied attitudes of doctors and patients about oral contraceptives and found
patchy consensus between doctor and patient attitudes. Doctors and
patients, he argued, should therefore be paired according to their com-
patibility in terms of how they structured meaning. This pluralistic and
technical approach to conditions of consensus stood in stark contrast to

the heated theological debates swirling around contraception use. Veatch tried to bridge the realms of logic and spirit, arguing that a turn to more "objective" discourse was still faithful to spiritual roots by providing an explanation for a realm of human experience difficult to account for—our ineffable (but palpably experienced) sense of purpose or belief. The experience of knowing something objectively, even if it took place within a specific context of meaning, strove to transcend the everyday. The experience of objectivity had, then, a "religious" quality: "Without the religious element of self-transcendence, of ultimate meaning, the objective command would not be felt."[73]

Moral aspects of medicine, which were once discussed almost exclusively by theologians, became the domain of secular professional ethicists. This aspect of the story of bioethics traces the transformation of the moral power of the sacred into the accessible tool of the philosopher or hospital ethics committee. It is not surprising that its formative figures were consciously seeking connections between their religious positions and new and exciting developments in academic moral philosophy, as well as in controversial and tumultuous social and political changes in the 1960s. Many of those controversies, such as those over contraception, abortion, and the newly blurred boundaries between life and death, focused on how to treat bodies. Veatch's path from divinity school to the secular domain paralleled that of bioethics as a whole, in the replacement of a theological tradition emphasizing discernible principles and rules by a secular philosophy with a similar emphasis on principles and rules. A vision of a secure, immanent moral universe shifted from God to the philosopher and, within medicine, from the doctor to the ethicist.

Accompanying this move to secular discourses and professional opportunities was a parallel debate over moral theology itself—should it emphasize the importance of rules or of context? This was not an abstract argument over the utility of different methods for moral theology, but was shaped by palpable social dislocation with respect to sexual norms, technological power, and the role of religious authority in 1950s and 1960s America. These arguments and this context were conveyed by the starkly different approaches to ethics taken by Paul Ramsey on the one hand, and by Beecher's friend Joseph Fletcher on the other.

We may never know for sure how carefully Beecher read the works of Fletcher, or of Moore, whom he also cited in *Research and the Individual*. But he regularly described himself in ways that incorporated the view of ethics that Fletcher advocated and that Veatch and Ramsey positioned themselves against. What divided Ramsey and Fletcher, and why is that relevant to talking about brain death? Ramsey was not hostile to the brain death criteria *per se*. His unease was outlined in the Lyman Beecher Lectures at Yale in 1969, which were published a year later as *The Patient as Person*. These reflected correspondence he'd had with Beecher expressing concern that the brain death definition meant that the heart would still have "spontaneous" capacity to beat in a "dead" person.[74] Either the criteria updated the definition of heart death in response to the inadequacy, revealed by artificial supports, of previous indicators of the heart's true death and loss of spontaneity. Or, the criteria suggested something quite different: a description of the primary importance of consciousness for descriptions of personhood. The latter violated respect for the sacredness of the body. Ramsey and others read a mixed message in the Report as to whether brain death was death because of lost capacity for consciousness or because of loss of spontaneous cardiopulmonary function. If tests of consciousness alone were the fundamental test of personhood, that would open the floodgates for opportunities to use patients as a means for the benefit of others.

Ramsey was also a widely read figure in debates through the 1960s about whether morality resulted from the set of relationships from within which a moral dilemma arose, or from reasoned rules and norms that guided and explained conduct.[75] Ramsey sided with the latter position. This dispute was in many ways a reprise of the Reformation conflict over grace versus deeds, over knowing what was right through one's own relationship with God versus following certain established values and rules. Ramsey feared ethics would lose, as its central consideration, *agape*, or Christian love, along with the demands *agape* placed on us. He also feared that reckless use of the idea of *agape* might only further a utilitarian, subjective morality. That is, one could expediently argue they were doing the "best" and most "loving" thing for another in order to justify any desired action. Rulemaking and rationality thus played a crucial, but particular, role for Ramsey—they helped avoid an "*agape* exceptionalism" and helped realize Christian love through rules that would structure moral choice.[76] Reflecting the tumult of sexual and political change in the 1960s—a common topic in these debates over rule/reason versus love/context ethics—he noted:

> Our contemporary penchant for escape-clauses and exception-making criteria to free the human spirit can only be compared with the displacement of sound political reason and statesmanship in the contemporary period by "crisis-manager" with their "rationality of irrationality" policies...In the absence of good *moral* reasoning, responsibility in moral action is reduced also to singular acts of the will...agape on one side, and quantifying reason on the other. Among men living in this hour the range of moral reason is considerably contracted. This explains why so many discover principle-less exceptions, both in personal morality and in social and political ethics.[77]

Ramsey sought a firm position on which to base rules faithful to *agape* in a pluralistic world. Mankind needed help and guidance to recognize and focus on *agape*, not freedom to individually craft it. One such firm position from which other rules could follow was the Christian commitment to the inviolability of the body, from which came his concern about a loss of consciousness-driven justification for brain death. Ramsey was wary of manipulating nature, and in particular of tampering with biological processes such as genetic endowment and reproduction for our own ends. His theology emphasized the sinfulness and limitations of man and the lack of capacity to exert significant dominion over nature. Ramsey's writings were deontological and skeptical of man's initiative with regard to God and nature. One contemporary critic described Ramsey's ethics as animated by an apocalyptic eschatology: The future held the likelihood that God would kill us all.[78]

Fletcher was among such critics and couldn't have been more different from Ramsey. His 1954 bestseller *Morals and Medicine*, and pretty much all that followed, celebrated human choice. Fletcher was on the side of those theologians who saw in history less the specter of the apocalypse than mankind's progressive and necessary engagement in shaping its own future. Technology held potential for great good. Choice over the fate of one's body was the true expression of humanity and the responsibilities that entailed. Sterilization, abortion, and euthanasia reflected appropriate legitimation of choices in the prerogatives of individuals, not in some moral code written in nature:

> A great deal of ethical reasoning in the past has been of this immoral kind—arguing against initiative and human control on grounds that it is allegedly "unnatural" or "against nature." That kind of ethics simply cannot survive in a technological civilization. "Nature" and "human nature" are no more fixed and finished than any of the other concepts moralists like to posit.[79]

Nor were decisions answerable to some static, unchanging notion of the holiness of the body that was blind to changes in how human agency could legitimately manipulate that body for the betterment and happiness of mankind:

> We are concerned primarily with man's spiritual quality and his selfhood. It is the integrity of the personality that has first claim in the forum of conscience. To be a person, to have a moral being, is to have the capacity for intelligent causal action. It means to be free of physiology!...But it is precisely persons—and not souls or bodies or glands or human biology—that count with God and come first in ethics.[80]

Fletcher's theological comfort with the prerogatives people had over their bodies allowed him to stake out a very different position from Ramsey in the raging norm-versus-context debate in American Christian moral theology. Fletcher, an Episcopalian minister, positioned himself within the work of such theologians as Reinhold Niebuhr, Martin Buber, and Dietrich Bonhoeffer. He saw in them as well the idea that moral theology focused attention on details rather than principles in moral situations, and that relationships with others shaped the nature and meaning of responsibility. This led Fletcher to emphasize that knowledge of what was moral in a given situation was attained through *agape*—a notable move in light of his oppositional stance toward Ramsey.

In a number of works, in particular *Moral Responsibility* and *Situation Ethics*.[81] Fletcher criticized what he saw as a dominance of a natural law tradition in particular and legalism in general in Christian moral theology. In contrast to Veatch or Ramsey, Fletcher saw himself more directly as *part* of a process, linked to Moore, that questioned the possibility of reifying or objectifying notions such as the "good." Good, justice, etcetera, were not properties at all. The goodness of an act lay in the very specific context in which it occurred and the motivations and results, in terms of *agape*, for those involved. Only within a specific effort to realize or sustain love—the only intrinsic good—could an act or belief of moral value be known. Fletcher repeated certain illustrative examples, such as a labor camp prisoner who purposefully became pregnant by a guard so as to be able to leave the camp and return home to her family. This was a moral act. Extramarital affairs, he argued in terms which were provocative at the time, could be considered moral if done in the context of a hopelessly loveless marriage and if motivated by the love and betterment of another in ways that otherwise respected the remaining marriage relationship.

Fletcher's position was a target of those concerned with what was often referred to as the "new morality." He was criticized for having an inconsistent notion of *agape*, for sending mixed messages about whether experience was best described in existential or theological terms, and for giving a morally unsatisfying account of how to use reason to apply *agape* to particular situations. But he also provided a rallying point for criticism of excessive legalism and naturalism in moral philosophy and theology, especially at a time of contested moral authority.[82]

Beecher's adoption of Fletcher's views deserves attention. They shared a perspective in which the ends determined the value and morality of

actions. "Indeed, unless justified by some end in view, any action is literally meaningless," wrote Fletcher.[83] Fletcher was unconcerned that a
renal dialysis committee might choose a mother of four over an alcoholic
to benefit from that scarce technology. Of course it would. As for brain
death, he was unconcerned with the physician moving in to usurp ultimate moral authority, to play God. Playing God was unavoidable; the
question was which God to play. Not the God of mystery and ignorance,
but of responsiveness to need.[84] A friend of Margaret Sanger, and labeled
the "Red Churchman" by Joseph McCarthy for his membership in the
Soviet-American Friendship Society among other things, Fletcher saw his
support of euthanasia, abortion, sterilization, and contraception as part of
a movement to free people from being "puppets." He is credited as a critical figure in shifting the justification of euthanasia from a eugenics-driven
rationale to one of moral choice and individual right.[85]

Beecher specifically endorsed Fletcher's situationalism. Moral action
was known deep within context, not reflectively outside of it, and that
required deep content knowledge of context, of medical facts and their
basis. Veatch and other critics endorsed opposing ideas about the nature
and purpose of moral facts, which in turn fit well with their efforts to
clarify, professionalize, and secularize expertise over physicians and their
increasingly dramatic interventions. Each, though, responded to the anxiety and mixed feelings about medicine's benefits and intrusions, and the
strangeness of embodiment that new technologies made hard to deny.

Beyond concepts and theory, the simple unsettling feeling that death
was being strangely moved ahead of dying was palpable among critics.
Leon Kass was a founding Fellow at Hastings and part of the initial work
there on death and dying that included the AAAS brain death panel and
published papers from it; he would later chair the Bioethics Council of
President George W. Bush. Kass corresponded with Beecher and acknowledged that while dying might be a continuous event, "this difficulty does
not warrant the conclusion that *death*, in contrast with *dying*, is a continuous event." Alongside his copy of these comments, Beecher wrote: "In our
fallible state we are unable to pinpoint death. We can only deal with the
process of dying and attempt to identify the state of no return."[86]

As Beecher argued in his marginalia and public comments, the content of the Harvard criteria initially came less from a drive for conceptual clarity than from the degree to which Schwab and his colleagues, as discussed further in Chapter Five, used (and needed) the criteria for those threshold situations when death was not distinguishable from dying in practice. In Eliasburg and *Research and the Individual*, Beecher reflected that medical dilemmas were dilemmas precisely because they pushed on the sensitive tensions between our biological and rights-bearing selves. An antidote to these dilemmas, then, needed a reliable broker of knowledge about the body. But while Beecher took much from Fletcher, Beecher's situationalism—as seen in his discussion of ends and means—was also positioned in a way that reflected the complexity of the space between Ramsey and Fletcher. *Agape* applied to physicians as well, and in that context it needed ground rules and specified responsibilities. Beecher considered science and medicine to be uniquely capable of engaging and solving core ethical challenges by virtue of how they managed the messy and contingent facts that were central for doing so. What was known and possible within the context of medical practice and knowledge could align means and ends.

In this way there was, in retrospect, a missed opportunity for a rich conversation between Beecher and Jonas that would have perhaps highlighted a different ethics dialogue around the purposes of medicine. Jonas's earlier work involved the history of Gnosticism; he described the transition from an ancient to a modern sensibility as a break from "the contention that the organic even in its lowest forms prefigures the mind, and that mind even in its highest reaches remains part of the organic." Both were essential and inseparable, according to Jonas: "A philosophy of life comprises the philosophy of the organism and the philosophy of mind."[87] Psychophysical unity was intrinsic to the meaning of "being." In a critique of his teacher Martin Heidegger's groundbreaking formulation of Being, a critique spurred by Jonas's disappointment in Heidegger's affiliation with Nazism, Jonas faulted the idealized distance of the existential point of view as the unsurprising result of that ancient–modern split which fueled a dangerous mind–body dualism. Such a dualism unmoored us from the organic world such that we saw nature as an inert "other" and a playground for our designs, rather than as a necessary source of values as it ought to be, Jonas argued, given our deep continuities with it:

> The living body that can die, that has world and itself belongs to the world, that feels itself and can be felt, whose outward form is organism and causality, and whose inward form is selfhood and finality; this body is the memento of the still unresolved question of ontology, "What is being?"[88]

Jonas found the scope of emerging technologies, especially in medicine, as an unprecedented "new kind of human action"[89] that was also a direct result of this dualism and permissive acting on nature as an object. Jonas saw in his quite different philosophy of life an answer to the question of where to find the needed brakes on this pace of change and manipulation of our being: "What force shall represent the future on the present? ... before the question of what *force*, comes the question of what *insight* or value-knowledge will represent the future in the present."[90]

For Beecher, medicine held the possibility for managing rather than wishing away the dualism Jonas faulted with unchecked assaults on our nature. Medicine was both a driver and, potentially, an antidote to this tendency toward technological manipulation of ourselves and the world. Beecher recognized this potential in the particular example of his limits around the respirator and in the weighing of ends and means. Beecher's challenge to Jonas to describe a path as to how to progress was one he thought medicine could answer. The perspective of medical work, immersed and generating knowledge from within the psychophysical unity, could bring Jonas's cosmic vision of mind's unified embeddedness in nature down to earth and more completely describe it. Medical knowledge and purpose were at the same time positioned to balance *that* fundamental, embedded, nature with the one that Jonas seemed to want to wish away: that is, the equally core feature of man to want to manipulate and even resist that nature.

Whatever dispute might be had with Beecher and his Committee, what clearly needs to be challenged is the historical characterization of their work as neither informed by, nor engaging with, thinking about ethics or the nature and purposes of medicine. A more sophisticated historical approach to these events, and to the history of medicine in general, can better explore how medical knowledge can and should mediate the dualism and ambivalence tied up with being embodied selves that suffer, but that don't want to.

NOTES

1. Henry Beecher, "The Right to be Let Alone; The Right to Die—Problems Created by the Hopelessly Unconscious Patient," The Fifth Bernard Eliasburg Memorial Lecture, Mount Sinai Hospital, New York City, December 6, 1967: Box 13, Folder 24, Beecher Papers. See Michael T. Kaufman, "Rights of a Man in Coma Pondered," *The New York Times*, Sunday, December 10, 1967. The annual Eliasberg Lecture began in 1963 to honor the first Chair of Anesthesiology at Mt. Sinai. Notable lecturers have included Nobel Prize recipient Linus Pauling.

2. Henry Beecher, "Ethical problems created by the hopelessly unconscious patient," *New England Journal of Medicine* 278, no. 26 (June 27, 1968): 1425–30.

3. Beecher, "The Right to be Let Alone," 1.

4. Edward A. Shils, "Social Inquiry and the Autonomy of the Individual," in *The Human Meaning of the Social Sciences*, ed. Daniel Lerner, (New York: Meridian Books, Inc., 1959), 114–57.

5. Shils, Ibid., 120, 118.

6. Eliasburg manuscript, 7.

7. Shils, "Social Inquiry," 121.

8. Ibid., 118.

9. Ibid., 8, 11.

10. See Beecher to Berry, June 6, 1965 and November 16, 1965, Box 6, Folder 71, Beecher Papers.

11. See typescript, "Notes for Report to Faculty of Medicine on Human Studies Committee," January 8, 1971, Box 6, Folder 85, Beecher Papers.

12. Henry K. Beecher, *Experimentation in Man* (Springfield, IL: Charles C. Thomas, 1958), and *Research and the Individual* (Boston: Little, Brown and Co., 1970). The first book appears to be essentially a reprint of a lengthy featured article in *JAMA* of the same title as a report by Beecher adopted by the American Medical Association Council on Drugs, and Committee on Research. Henry Beecher, "Experimentation in man," *JAMA* 169 (1959): 461–78.

13. Henry K. Beecher, *Measurement of Subjective Responses: Quantitative Effects of Drugs* (New York: Oxford University Press, 1959).

14. Beecher, *Research and the Individual*, 24, 26.

15. Henry Beecher, "The powerful placebo," *JAMA* 159, no. 17 (December 24, 1955): 1602–6, 1606.

16. Henry Beecher, "Experimentation in man," 470.

17. Ibid., 473.

18. Henry Beecher, *Research and the Individual* (Boston: Little, Brown, 1970).

19. Henry Beecher, "Consent in clinical experimentation in man: myth and reality," *JAMA* 195, no. 1 (January 3, 1966): 34–35. Henry Beecher, "Some fallacies and errors in the application of the principle of informed consent," *Clinical Pharmacology and Therapeutics* 3 (March–April 1962): 141–45.

20. Beecher, *Research and the Individual*, 20.

21. Ibid., 23, 26.

22. Minutes, Human Studies Committee, Box 8, Folder 63, Beecher Papers.

23. For an interpretation of controversy over the acceptability of controlled trials as a story of the socialization of standardization over individual judgments, see Theodore Porter, *Trust in Numbers* (Princeton: Princeton University Press, 1995). For other historical forces shaping consensus around experimental methods for controlled and randomized methods for proving efficacy, Ted J. Kaptchuk, "Intentional ignorance: a history of blind assessment and placebo controls in medicine," *Bulletin of the History of Medicine* 72, no. 3 (Fall 1998): 389–433.

24. Henry Beecher, "Some guiding principles of clinical investigation," *JAMA* 195, no. 13 (March 28, 1966): 1135–36, 1135.

25. Benjamin Freedman, "Equipoise and the ethics of clinical research," *The New England Journal of Medicine* 317, no. 3 (1987): 141–45. For some indications of the subsequent debate surrounding this idea see Franklin G. Miller and Howard Brody, "A critique of clinical equipoise: therapeutic misconception in the ethics of clinical trials," *The Hastings Center Report* 33, no. 3, (2003): 19–28, and Robert Veatch, "The irrelevance of equipoise," *Journal of Medical Philosophy* 32, no. 2 (2007): 167–83. Criticisms include that equipoise generally takes the point of view of physicians or researchers, not the subjects for whom determination of the equal positions of treatment options may or may not be shared. Similarly, looking at research from a balance of clinical benefit implied a therapeutic relationship between the researcher and the subject that risked a therapeutic misconception. That is, subjects could mistakenly understand their participation in research to be treatment, and thus were vulnerable in terms of motives for participation and misunderstanding of risks. See my historical perspective on—and critique of—this "misconception" in Gary S. Belkin, "Misconceived bioethics? The misconception of the therapeutic 'misconception,'" *International Journal of Law and Psychiatry* 29 (2006): 75–85. The issues Beecher explored remain a relevant part of a tension over what drives physician obligations to subjects.

26. R. L. Addinall, "Cowardly patient," *Science* 153 (August 12, 1966): 694.

27. Beecher, *Research and the Individual*, 27–29.

28. Beecher to Berry, May 28, 1965, Box 6, Folder 16, Beecher Papers.

29. Henry Beecher and Donald P. Todd, " A study of the deaths associated with anesthesia and surgery," *Annals of Surgery* (1954): 140.

30. Beecher, Typescript of Address at Central Connecticut State College, Oct 19, 1966, Box 30, Folder 33, Beecher Papers, 16.

31. Beecher's main source for this was the prolific author and science commentator, Bentley Glass, *Science and Ethical Values* (Chapel Hill: University of North Carolina Press, 1965).

32. Beecher, *Research and the Individual*, 206.

33. Fletcher to Beecher, March 20, 1971, Box 11, Folder 24, Beecher Papers.

34. Beecher, *Research and the Individual*, 211.

35. Ibid., 211–12.

36. This reflected as well the position at the time of the Board of Medicine of the National Academy of Sciences, which issued a statement specifically about cardiac transplantation making clear that such a procedure should be regarded as research. "The ethical issues involved...are a part of the whole complex question of the ethics of human experimentation." Board on Medicine, National Academy of Sciences, "Cardiac transplantation in man," *JAMA* 204, no. 9, (May 1968): 147–48, 148. It is worth remembering that skepticism about heart transplantation ran high. As one *JAMA* editorial put it: "transplantation of the heart cannot survive as a valid procedure," doubting with unveiled sarcasm that a supply of hearts could not exist without new coercions. See "Have a heart," *JAMA* 203, no. 5 (Jan. 29, 1968): 356–57, 356. See also "The sky watchers," *JAMA* 204, no. 9 (May 27, 1968): 820–21. There, the editors stated they were "unconvinced of the merits of heart transplantation" (821).

37. Henry Beecher, "The New Definitions of Death, Some Opposing Views," manuscript, 1971, Box 16, Folder 18, Beecher Papers, 5.

38. Robert M. Veatch, "Brain death: welcome definition or dangerous judgment?," *Hastings Center Report* (November 1972): 10–13, 10–11.

39. Robert M. Veatch, "Remarks on Dr. Henry K. Beecher's Paper 'The New Definitions of Death, Some Opposing Views,'" AAAS Chicago, Box 16, Folder 18, Beecher Papers, 6.

40. See *Death, Dying and the Biological Revolution: Our Last Quest for Responsibility* (New Haven: Yale University Press, 1976). Veatch continued to argue this scheme in later writings over subsequent decades.

41. Robert M. Veatch, "Remarks on Dr. Henry K. Beecher's Paper," 4.

42. Jonsen in particular characterizes this address as shattering the isolation of medicine from proper philosophical study, describing it as "a landmark in the ethics of experimentation and in bioethics in general...Hans Jonas gave to the ethics of research a solid philosophical foundation," Jonsen, *The Birth of Bioethics*, 150–51.

43. Hans Jonas, "Philosophical reflections on human experimentation," in *Daedalus: Ethical Aspects of Experimentation with Human Beings* (Spring 1969): 219–47, 227.

44. Ibid., 230.

45. Ibid., 228.

46. Henry Beecher, "The new definition of death. Some opposing views," *International Journal of Clinical Pharmacology, Therapy and Toxicology* 5, no. 2 (April 14, 1971): 120–24, 123. This paper approximates the manuscript version of the same title cited above, to have been presented at AAAS, which Veatch and Ramsey criticize.

47. Ibid., 122. Jonsen's *Birth of Bioethics* sets up physician Walsh McDermott's argu-
    ment that the good of society can trump the rights of some individuals when it
    comes to experimentation as Jonas's target. This philosopher–physician opposition
    is critical to Jonsen's narrative of the unique, needed, and valuable expertise of
    bioethics philosophers. But Beecher's own concerns and cautions about societal
    claims also complicates both Jonas's and Jonsen's use of this narrative.
48. Beecher marginalia on manuscript copy of Paul Ramsey, "Comment on 'The New
    Definition of Death, Some Opposing Views,' by Henry K. Beecher," Box 16 Folder
    16, Beecher Papers, 4.
49. Ibid., 7.
50. Ibid., 5.
51. Daniel Callahan, *The Roots of Bioethics: Health, Progress, Technology, Death*
    (New York: Oxford University Press, 2012).
52. Henry Beecher, "The new definition of death. Some opposing views."
53. Robert Veatch, "Whole-brain, neocortical, and higher brain-related concepts."
54. Robert M. Veatch, "Remarks on Dr. Henry K. Beecher's Paper," 2.
55. Ibid., 7.
56. Veatch, "Remarks on Dr. Henry K. Beecher's Paper," 1.
57. Ibid., 4.
58. Beecher, typescript, "Notes for Report to Faculty of Medicine on Human Studies
    Committee," 3, January 8, 1971, Box 6, Folder 85, Beecher Papers.
59. Ibid., 4.
60. Ibid., 12.
61. Ibid., 1.
62. Henry Beecher, "Some moral and ethical problems confronting the medical inves-
    tigator," Old South Church on the occasion of its 300th anniversary, Feb 9, 1969,
    Box 12, Folder 32, Beecher Papers, 16.
63. Ramsey, "Comment on 'The New Definition of Death, Some Opposing Views,' by
    Henry K. Beecher," Box 16 Folder 16, Beecher Papers, 4.
64. Roderick Firth, "Ethical absolutism and the ideal observer," *Philosophy and
    Phenomenological Research* 12, no. 3 (March 1952, 12): 317–45, 319.
65. G. E. Moore, *Principia Ethica* (Cambridge: Cambridge University Press, 1991
    [1903]). See especially 10–17.
66. William Frankena, *Ethics* (Englewood Cliffs, NJ: Prentice-Hall, 1963).
67. Veatch specifically acknowledged his reliance upon Firth and Rawls as singular
    influences. See Jonsen, *Birth of Bioethics,* 56–57.
68. Robert M. Veatch, "Medical ethics: professional or universal?," *Harvard Theological
    Review* 65 (1972): 531–59.
69. See for example Callahan's collection of essays that addresses the necessity of
    Catholic intellectual inclusion in mainstream forms of inquiry, *The New Church*
    (New York: Charles Scribner's Sons, 1966), and his book on abortion, below.
70. Daniel Callahan, *Abortion: Law, Choice and Morality* (New York: The Macmillan
    Co., 1970).
71. Daniel Callahan, "The Sanctity of Life," in *Updating Life and Death*, ed. Donald
    R. Cutler (Boston: Beacon Press, 1969): 181–223.

72. Daniel Callahan, "Response," 243–50, 250.

73. Veatch, *Value Freedom*, 111.

74. Paul Ramsey, *The Patient as Person* (New Haven: Yale University, 1970). See especially Chapter Two, "On Updating Procedures for Stating that a Man Has Died," 59–112.

75. Paul Ramsey, *Deeds and Rules in Christian Ethics* (New York: Charles Scribners Sons, 1967), Gene Outka, Paul Ramsey, eds., *Norm and Context in Christian Ethics* (New York: Charles Scribner's Sons, 1968), Charles E. Curran, ed., *Absolutes in Moral Theology?* (Washington: Corpus Books, 1968).

76. Paul Ramsey, "The Case of the Curious Exception," in *Norm and Context in Christian Ethics*, eds. Gene Outka, Paul Ramsey, 67–135.

77. Ibid., 93.

78. For this view of Ramsey, as well as a good entree to this natural law debate, see Charles C. Curran, *Contemporary Problems in Moral Theology* (Notre Dame, IN: Fides Publisher, Inc., 1970).

79. Joseph Fletcher, "Technological devices in medical care," in *Who shall live? Medicine, Technology, Ethics*, ed. Kenneth Vaux (Philadelphia: Fortress Press, 1970): 116–42, 124.

80. Joseph Fletcher, *Morals and Medicine* (Boston: Beacon Press, 1954): 218–19.

81. Joseph Fletcher, *Moral Responsibility, Situation Ethics at Work* (Philadelphia: The Westminster Press, 1967); *Situation Ethics: The New Morality* (Philadelphia: The Westminster Press, 1966).

82. For a collection of responses to Fletcher's *Situation Ethics* and its place in the broader debate within moral theology, see Harvey Cox, ed., *The Situation Ethics Debate* (Philadelphia: Westminster Press, 1968).

83. Fletcher, *Moral Responsibility*, 22.

84. Joseph Fletcher, "On Death," in *Updating Life and Death*, ed. Donald R. Cutler (Boston: Beacon Press, 1969).

85. Ian Dowbiggin, *A Merciful End: The Euthanasia Movement in Modern America* (New York: Oxford University Press, 2002), 100–102.

86. Kass to Beecher, May 20, 1970, Box 16, Folder 12, Beecher Papers.

87. Hans Jonas, *The Phenomenon of Life: Towards a Philosophical Biology* (Evanston, IL: Northwestern University Press, 2001 [1966]), 1.

88. Ibid., 19.

89. Hans Jonas, *The Imperative of Responsibility: In Search of an Ethics for the Technological Age* (Chicago: University of Chicago Press, 1984), 23.

90. Ibid., 22.

3

The Law

"We take judicial notice that one breathing, though unconscious, is not dead."
—SMITH V. SMITH, *1958*

"The extraordinary definition of death is tending toward recognition of "life" as neurological in form, and that an interruption of the cerebral function should be the determining point in deciding that death is present, regardless of the continued function of other organs."
—M. MARTIN HALLEY AND WILLIAM HARVEY,
Indiana Legal Forum, 1968

The differences between Beecher's Committee and its critics over what sort of fact death should be, as discussed in the prior chapter, reflected a tangle over what were actually shared problems that could not easily or most usefully be reduced to a contest between ethics and medicine. Rather, such conflicts arose from differing experiences with ethical and medical facts. Self-described ethicists were not the only ones concerned about whether death was properly framed as a fact by medical practice. Lawyers and judges were also explicitly concerned with what kind of fact death was, and with what concepts and experiences were relevant to its definition. They tended to consider these issues with a pragmatism that was similar to that of Beecher and the Committee.

William Curran's job was to address the legal standing of death based on irreversible coma. Beecher circulated an early draft of Curran's section of the Report to Committee members in April 1968. It was a verbatim reproduction of "Notes" Curran had prepared apparently for the Committee meeting of March 14.[1] The task of that section, as it finally appeared in the published Report, was to argue that there was legal sanction for the shift from regarding breathing and circulation as the fundamental signs of life, to the "recognition of 'life' as neurological in form," and, furthermore, "that an interruption of the cerebral function should be the determining point in deciding that death is present."[2]

The legal authority for such a shift was not obviously supported in the Report. Courts had regularly referred, mantra-like, to the authoritative *Black's Law Dictionary*, which specified the loss of respiration, circulation, and pulsation as the definition of death. Case law that had ventured into the question of when death occurred had relied on that description of the end of life for decades, if not centuries. But a shift, the Report argued, was not as exceptional as it appeared, because the durable principle in *Black's* was itself less about lungs and hearts than about how the judiciary generally deferred to medical consensus. The law, the Report asserted, would adopt shifts in medical opinion and in the conditions of medical practice. Others argued that as well. And essentially that is what happened.

Interpreting this shift merely as an example of "medicalization," as most commentators have, can deter curiosity as to how this change happened— from defining life as breathing and beating to "neurological in form"—and exactly what was changing in this process. While judicial (and legislative) deference to medical judgment was certainly the overall trend in the case of defining death, the motor of that trend was arguably more than simply the power of physicians or medically defined ends. The increasing adoption of a view of ourselves as "neurobiological selves" over the past half-century is too superficially laid at the feet of assertive medical professionals. A confluence of larger conceptual, economic, technological, and biopolitical changes are needed to explain this change, one that carries risks of objectification, but also possibilities to enrich and accelerate social, medical, and ethical ways of knowing.[3] Early in this shift toward a more neurological definition of death, before the criteria appeared several legal scholars called for such reconsideration of how to define death. The intrusion of medicine-speak into judicial fact finding has always had complex purposes and results. It could advance democratization and empowerment in fact finding, but could also increase reliance on expert authority.[4] Where was legal opinion on brain death coming from?

CURRAN'S NOTES

In his "Notes," Curran reviewed "the few modern court decisions involving a definition of death." He detailed three cases, widely described in legal medicine circles, in which there was a question as to the relative timing of death of two persons who died in the same accident, or as to the cause of death when kidneys were removed from a "brain dead" individual. Should a woman be considered to have died after her husband, given the fact that her death was declared at the time of cardiac arrest while unconscious on a respirator some time after the accident that also "instantly" killed him? Did a man die when his breathing spontaneously ceased? Or, when subsequently placed on a respirator, was it the later removal of both of his kidneys for transplant that claimed his life?[5]

Curran selected cases that closely matched the facts of brain death so as to anticipate judicial response to the use of the Report's criteria. These cases involved people whose conditions resembled the ones that the Committee was trying to define. Several physicians instrumental in establishing the biology and care of the severely comatose, such as Fred Plum, C. Miller Fischer, and several of their contemporaries (whose work I will explore further) had been making decisions to turn off respirators at least since the latter 1950s without recalling significant concern at the time for legal barriers or lawsuit.[6] What role, then, did this review of legal cases play in the Report?

Curran's memorandum predicted what to expect from a judge if the brain death criteria were brought before a court. Not surprisingly, Curran found that no precedent existed for legal recognition of brain death. What he found were cases that, despite the appearance of factual similarities, did not directly address the relevant issues. Much of Curran's memorandum explained how these cases presented legal questions not directly germane to what he saw as the question facing the Committee; that is, whether brain death would be recognized within the common law as death. The inquest case, for example, was widely quoted, as it seemed perhaps the only case up to that time to rule on the legal validity of brain death. In that case, a man who was knocked unconscious in a fight was brought to the hospital, placed on a respirator, and determined unsalvageable due to brain injury. His wife gave permission to remove his kidneys for the purpose of transplantation. They were removed and then the respirator turned off. A coroner's inquest found that the cause of death was the original injury, not the kidney removal. But it was unlikely that this case offered a reliable precedent to support use of the brain death criteria. As Curran pointed out in his memorandum, a coroner's jury could not make law and, more to the point, the legal issue in this case was the cause, not the criteria, of death. The surgeon was found not to have changed the outcome. Indeed, if any criteria of death were endorsed in this case, it was that of the loss of heart-lung function, since doctors testified that the patient was already dead, as in not breathing, before being placed on the respirator. He died first. This logic set up precisely the dilemma that concerned the Committee and that the inquest thought it avoided—namely that by relying on that traditional definition, logical consistency required that this individual be understood to have been reanimated, brought *back* to life when put on the respirator, a point which contradicted the premise that the surgeon did not cause the death. The inquest offered no legal clarity for this dilemma, despite the apparent opportunity to do so. It may have instead opened the door to further confusion.

The two simultaneous death cases Curran cited were, similarly, not directly germane to the legal legitimacy of brain death. *Smith v. Smith* received most of Curran's attention because the opinion explicitly endorsed the notion that one who is "breathing, though unconscious, is not dead."[7] That opinion would appear to reject brain death. But the legal significance of this statement, Curran opined, was not as it appeared.

The judge in *Smith* took "judicial notice" that continued breathing ruled out death, meaning that he described death as a fact enjoying a consensus such that he would not entertain evidence to the contrary. "Consensus" generally meant the *Black's Law Dictionary's* definition of death as a "total stoppage of the circulation of the blood" and a "cessation of the animal and vital spirits consequent thereupon, such as respiration, pulsation, etc."[8] But Curran explained that the "notice" was less a ruling on one definition as opposed to others than it was a statement to the effect that the law assumed there was a background consensus as to what criteria for death were. These near-miss judicial encounters with brain death led Curran to conclude that there was a pervasive legal attitude that death had a settled definition and was not controversial. It was a biological fact, with a broad consensus. Most of this analysis remained in the final Report.

But in the legal section, the Report included three closing paragraphs that were not found in Curran's original draft, and that took a direction Curran did not originally go. Pushing Curran's point about consensus, the Report essentially argued that legal notice could be won for a new definition if it reflected a new consensus. Acknowledging the frequent deference to the *Black's* definition, the Report continued:

> In this report, however, we suggest that responsible medical opinion is ready to adopt new criteria for pronouncing death to have occurred in an individual sustaining irreversible coma as a result of permanent brain damage. If this position is adopted by the medical community, it can form the basis for change in the current legal concept of death.[9]

Since prior cases had not ruled on the specific question the Committee was asking, the Committee chose to interpret widespread deference to *Black's* as a reflection of the way courts generally *approached* the issue of the definition of death, rather than a commitment specifically to the heart/lung functioning enshrined in *Black's*. The cases were used to conclude that when it came to defining death, courts were concerned with process (to acknowledge settled background consensus on this fact of biology as consensus developed), rather than specific content (to acknowledge only heart-lung definitions or concepts). Judges wanted to know if there was a clear consensus, not what that consensus was.

This emphasis on arguing for a new background consensus was different from Curran's original idea. The background consensus, after all, *was* one of a heart-beating-and-breathing notion of death, so a change had to have a legal reason other than that some people had changed their minds. So, Curran's initial advice for how to effect change was not to appeal to the authority of a new background consensus but to seek the recognition and leeway that courts often gave to the adaptation of legal definitions when faced with markedly changed circumstances, needs, and consequences.

Why did the Committee choose the change-of-consensus route, rather than the changed-circumstances approach that was initially proposed by its lawyer? Curran, for his part, referred in the Notes to growing legal commentary over the conflict between transplantation and existing statutes. He considered this a major part of the new needs and consequences for which brain death represented a response. Curran advised that broaching such conflicts would require more than redefining death in terms of brain death. Death definitions, however derived, could resolve only some legal problems of transplantation. The law left large holes that medical consensus on the definition of death—and legal recognition of the controlling authority of such consensus—would not fill:

> The question before this committee cannot be simply to define brain death. This would not advance the cause of organ transplantation since it would not cope with the essential issue of when the surgical team is authorized...in removing a vital organ. It would not, of itself, answer the question of when there is justification (in whom?) to turn off the respirator. It also does not cope with the question of the reason for placing the person on the respirator in the first place. Separate issues of law are raised by all of these questions...Courts of law will not be satisfied to find that definitions of terms prepared for other purposes and under other assumptions are being used to prevent the saving of lives without preserving other important values. The conflicting

values here may be the "vegetable existence" of one person as against the full life of another. The courts may well be willing to find greater value in saving the life of the one. A deeper analysis of the meaning of life seems to me necessary here. This deeper meaning would be concerned with the *quality of life*, not mere "existence," which is the key term in the definitions in the law dictionaries...of the values which make human existence worthwhile and tolerable this side of the veil of tears.[10]

Curran invited the Committee to delve into a comprehensive agenda needed to advance and respond to a range of new medical practices, and to describe norms for justified treatment withdrawal more broadly.

This direction was not taken. In correspondence with Beecher following review of his initial draft, Curran acknowledged that the Committee's consensus called for a more narrowed task, and thus that his draft "should not be included. It was prepared only as background."[11] Rather than argue and comprehensively address the ways that meanings of life and imperatives for transplantation had changed—and, consequently, the ways that judicial logic ought to change as well—the Report would identify a change in medical logic and conditions of care that deserved judicial notice. Curran agreed his section would therefore focus on the more restricted purview likely settled on after the meeting, as outlined in this letter to Beecher:

(1) A complete and comprehensive set of guidelines for the determination of irreversible brain damage...(2) Guidelines and procedures for the handling of such persons on respirators and other extraordinary means of prolonging life. It may also be necessary for us to make suggestions concerning the "certifying" of death and the signing of death certificates.[12]

Curran's draft of the legal section underwent the most revisions and was explicitly edited to argue that while the definition of irreversible coma itself couldn't (and shouldn't) resolve decisions about handling the body for the purposes of transplantation, the definition *could* in and of itself clarify a medical consensus on the nature and consequences of this type of coma.

Thus the Report concluded that "responsible medical opinion was ready to adopt new criteria for pronouncing death to have occurred in an individual sustaining irreversible coma." This conclusion empowered physicians to "declare the person dead, and then turn off the respirator."[13] Curran's initial advisement that the definition alone would not justify turning off the respirator was resisted in the final Report. The Report also described an assumed protective power of "shared responsibility," despite Curran's skepticism in this matter. Curran shared with Beecher a criticism of a paper by Schwab and Rosoff, that argued that shared responsibility by more than one physician when declaring brain death would offer legal protection.[14] Curran wrote Beecher that "I really don't see how they could 'share' his legal responsibility by consultation."[15] But the Report drew the opposite conclusion.

The final Report, in Curran's eyes, could not have resolved the issues surrounding transplantation. It severely stretched, if not broke, much of his original advice and purposes. The Report's editorial choices instead underscored a narrower focus on the issue of cessation of brain function and how this affected the ways in which doctors performed their recognized task of declaring death. In one of the most widely quoted sentences to appear in later newspaper descriptions, the Report emphasized that "no statutory change in the law should be necessary since the law treats this question essentially as one of fact determined by physicians."[16] The implications of this conclusion would follow in due course, but not in the Report or by the Committee. The Report more closely resembled the Schwab paper that Curran criticized. Schwab's concern was not transplant, or the meaning of life, but generally recognizing that removing care from an artificially maintained corpse be seen for what it was, and not be mistaken as an action causing death.

Two aspects of legal opinion up until the late 1960s are worth reviewing here in some further detail, as they underscore the Committee's purpose to describe the consequences of neurological death, rather than to write policy to facilitate transplant. The first aspect was how the

Report's conclusion about the significance of a new medical consensus compared with the body of case law that was selectively represented by Curran. The second was how other legal literature and opinion engaged these issues.

TIMING DEATH

The two simultaneous death cases explored by Curran were a very small sampling of a rather large volume of legal opinion that addressed how to determine the timing of death. *Smith v. Smith* was a relatively late addition to a thick fabric of judicial reasoning over disputes as to whether two deaths did or did not occur simultaneously. Resolution of such disputes over timing was often critical for the purposes of determining the disposition of wills and property. Curran correctly saw in *Smith* no ruling on the specific question of the validity of brain death. He and the Committee instead emphasized how the case spoke to the kinds of authority and evidence used by courts to determine the time of death. These cases, then, provide some access to how evidence and facts were used in legal proceedings to describe death before 1968.

When Hugh and Lucy Coleman Smith had a car accident while driving together on April 19, 1957, Hugh was considered dead at the scene, but Lucy remained "unconscious" in a coma for seventeen days until she "died." Both had prepared wills that bequeathed their estates, and the executor functions of those estates, to each other. Petitioners asked the court to construct the wills since they died simultaneously. The court denied the request. The court's opinion joined this case to a tradition of other cases dealing with the methods and burdens of proof necessary for a finding of simultaneous death. State and local courts frequently reviewed situations in which joint deaths of spouses or of parents with their children occurred and, further, in which the precise sequence of those deaths was often crucial to how a will and associated property were disposed. By the time the Smiths died, at least thirty-seven states had adopted some form of the Uniform Simultaneous Death Act of the National Conference of Commissioners on Uniform State Laws. This Act was developed to address such dilemmas, and significant case law had emerged to interpret those statutes.

Interpretations turned on how to define the burden of proof needed to show that deaths were simultaneous. State laws included various versions of language from the Uniform Act that approached the problem in a negative way. That is, if there was "no sufficient evidence" that the deaths were *other* than simultaneous, then they would be assumed to be simultaneous. Depending on how stringently this sufficient evidence standard was construed by courts, or redefined by some state legislatures, the burden for finding nonsimultaneity ranged between needing to prove simultaneity or, conversely, needing to assume and then disprove it. The opinion in *Smith v. Smith* clarified the sufficient evidence standard for proof in Arkansas. In doing so, this case and similar others provide a revealing look at judicial understanding of the practice and evidence for defining death.

A patient who was "breathing, though unconscious, is not dead,"[17] argued the opinion. While Curran took pains to underscore such a conclusion as procedural—that is, as clarifying the process for determining simultaneity—the opinion revealed clear assumptions on the part of the judiciary about what constituted relevant evidence. The opinion in *Smith v. Smith* went to great lengths to cite case law that accepted the authority of "common sense" in making such determinations. The court found that it stretched such sense to say that Mrs. Smith, though without consciousness and thus "power to will," could still be "breathing" yet at the same time be considered dead as of the onset of her unconsciousness, as petitioners claimed. The court characterized this claim as "a quite unusual and unique allegation."[18] The petitioners added to this confusion by originally arguing that before Mrs. Smith "died," she had since "remained in a coma" and, further, that it would "probably be several months before she would be considered competent." Thus, the petitioners argued, an appointed estate administrator was necessary until "she will be able...to manage her own affairs."[19] First she was described by her attorneys as temporarily incompetent but very much alive, while weeks later they argued that she had been dead all along. Common sense was indeed offended.

In a world of death before dying, a world that Curran and his colleagues were starting to create and inhabit, this construction was not surprising. But in case law and the very tangible and consequential sorts of problems it tried to order and characterize, it was. An indication of this breach in experience was that, in several places, the opinion described the patient as "breathing." In a 1968 presentation at an American Neurological Association (ANA) meeting, Schwab described this court case and stated that Mrs. Smith was supported by a respirator.[20] Given the timing of the ANA meeting (at which Schwab announced that the Ad Hoc Committee was still deliberating), it is most likely that Schwab's knowledge of the case came from Curran and his Notes. However, Curran's summary of the case did not suggest that the patient was on a respirator but instead used the word "breathing" as used in the opinion. The opinion itself made no such reference to a respirator, only to breathing. The question of which characterization was correct is as interesting as the confusion itself. If the patient was indeed on a respirator, then the opinion regarded this circumstance as no different than usual "breathing." If not, then possibly Curran, or more likely Schwab, upon reading about the case, interpreted "breathing" to mean a respirator, or simply assumed that she required a respirator. "Breathing" contained newly murky meanings and projections that could be associated with no voluntary or independent action but still mark relevant, human, estate-owning life. On the other hand, breathing could be assumed to describe a spurious artifice in a dead body.

The judicial review of the contested wills of Otho and Lois Pierce in *Schmitt vs Pierce* was one of a host of cases further detailing this gap between case law and the experiences of some physicians as to the consequences of the persisting mechanics of the body. "The collision occurred about 1:05 p.m. on a cold day, about 10 miles south of Poplar Bluff on Highway 53."[21] This was the second marriage for both Pierces, and each had children with their prior spouse. They had each bequeathed portions of their estate to their respective children, as well as to each other. Who died first was important as it determined whose estate was transferred to whom. Parsing prior case law and the Uniform Act, the court reviewed the burden of evidence necessary to find that the deaths had not occurred simultaneously. What is particularly worth highlighting about this case and about many other simultaneity rulings was the evidence itself: "Link testified Mrs. Pierce was bleeding from the ears before they moved her, and he distinctly heard her moan or groan, when they moved her, Barker and Wilburn each…did not hear Mrs. Pierce moan or groan while moving her."[22] Link and Mrs. Metcalf saw blood pumping from her ears; Bridewell said it would "ooze"; some witnesses described a "trickle"; still others saw only "a little dry blood." Barker recalled holding her head and stating, "'she is gone,'" as Trooper Link stood over him, nodding his head in agreement. And yet, according to the case "Link did not remember this." Clark said her eyes were open, "'with a glare look'"; Mrs. Davis that they were closed; and Mr. Davis took the moderate path and said that they were "open a little bit; not too much." Some saw regularly changing bloody air bubbles getting larger and smaller, and bursting about the nose; another did not observe Mrs. Pierce breathing but said that "she did gasp in a manner a person still breathing would." Mr. Askew observed "some kind of movement, 'enough to notice it.'" Mrs. Pierce's pulse was not taken. Mr. Pierce had dried blood and no movement. He had no pulse in the car. "He was lying there lifeless."[23]

Expert medical testimony argued that all these movements described in Mrs. Pierce could have been present in a dead body as the result of collapsed blood vessels, expiration of air by collapsing lungs, and the final twitches of muscles. The mélange of disorganized gurglings, oozings, and movements had to be organized coherently by the court. As with the Smiths' deaths and numerous other cases, this kind of information was sifted to balance the legal status of "common sense" on the question of defining death on the one hand, and the burden of sufficiency of evidence to negate simultaneity on the other. Expert medical testimony in this particular case took a back seat to the "common sense" of movement and blood. Despite inconsistent and conflicting renderings, blood was there, physically moving, as Black's quoted definition seemed to emphasize. The opinion concluded that "the trial court could find plaintiffs met the burden resting upon them by substantial evidence of survivorship."[24]

The status of background expert opinion in these cases seemed far less dominant or certain than Curran and the Committee concluded it was. As one court found, whether someone appeared dead or alive was "something within the common knowledge of mankind." Expert testimony insisted on the need for a stethoscope to determine death, since lack of movement or variable pulse or sounds from a body could be misleading. But that insistence did not sway the court's confidence in a lay witness's conclusions, formed from visual impression at a distance by lantern-light and "based on his having previously seen dead people."[25] There was, as Curran stated, a general background consensus as to what death was. But whatever deference judges gave to "background consensus," that consensus was not commonly attributed to physicians or their expertise. The *Black's* definition, while frequently quoted, was rarely engaged as a definition, as this definition itself was vague and contradictory, and was used in different ways. With a clarity reminiscent of the well known "duck" of obscenity, the judiciary in this case did not need to establish a formal definition or attempt to parse a definition out in order to recognize death when they saw it.

When courts did turn to physicians, they often did so in ways that reinforced the semiotics of movement, flow, and blood. In one case, a couple was run over by a train. Physicians argued that the primary importance of blood flow and movement led to the conclusion that wife survived husband because a witness saw spurts of blood from the site of her decapitated head, but not from his more intact body. Her body was not dead as long as the heart beat, even though her head was completely severed.[26] This interpretation of physical signs could locate and justify, in an apparent one-second difference between two deaths, space enough for the transfer of an estate.[27] A child's gurglings for a one- to two-minute period right after birth met the burden to prove its survivorship.[28] A feeling of warmth to the touch and some minutes of persistent breathing could satisfy a burden of proof for survivorship of one body beyond that of a cool fellow victim in a house fire, despite that fact that the latter received artificial respiration.[29]

While there seemed to be a backdrop of consensus, when death was revealed in its particulars in these legal rulings it was shown to be tightly connected to the whirring and color of the body. This backdrop of consensus was not founded in consciousness, or even in actual confirmed heart or lung functioning. This is not to say that the issue of consciousness wasn't debated. A draft of the Uniform Simultaneous Death Act report-edly specified that "a priority of time shall not be deemed to be suffi-ciently evidenced unless [during] such an interval of time between the deaths is shown to have elapsed . . . the survivor had a clear period of con-sciousness."[30] But this provision—which potentially introduced the idea of the capacity for consciousness as a factor in timing of death—was not adopted as standard. Physical movement and tangible signs, accessible to "the common man" and consistent with centuries of practice in listening and looking for movement, were the preferred tools.

Quite different from this standard, and more commonly used on hospi-tal wards, was an alternative understanding of the body—one that instead highlighted the functions of its brain and its capacity for consciousness. The differences between these approaches to understanding life or death lay in experiences more than in clear descriptions or concepts. As con-cepts, these approaches were much more easily reconciled. But as experi-ences, the emotional, tactile, and practical tasks presented by each were farther apart. One experience was physical, palpable, textured, and col-ored, closely identifying the superficial appearances of the mangled body with its humanity. The other was in some ways more distant from the emo-tion and meaning stirred by the physical changes and dynamism of the body. But in other ways, this second type of experience provided a more penetrating way to search for possible awareness, communication, and engagement—to search, in essence, for deeper and less overt evidences of physiological capacity using specific planned provocations of the nervous system in search of a patterned response.

These were, and are, differences not readily reduced to definition. The concept of either brain death or of a circulatory, heart/lung death made sense first depending upon the adequacy with which it joined an experi-ence of the body to relevant circumstances. Brain death became a work-able and "obvious" concept within and because of the conditions of death before dying. Under these conditions death was comprehensible as a dynamic category that could be suspended, considered. The movement from person to corpse became more elaborately negotiated and managed, such that the presence of death preceded dying.

New hospital practices meant changes in the experienced signs of life and death, signs that would move death determination further away from the view of the "common man." On several occasions Beecher noted that any change in consensus required broader social agreement and confidence. In subsequent writings and talks, he stressed how physician consensus on defining death as brain death required public acceptance in order to work and be legitimate. Even if courts were to acknowledge this new practice, it might avoid the need for statute but not the need for broad consensus. The Report offered criteria around which to build that consensus. And in law journals and proliferating panels and forums, there are some signs of just such a point of view beginning to appear among legal scholars in the 1950s and 1960s. In part as a response to address the new and growing gap between the medical and case law experiences of the dying body, these ideas—that death criteria were a matter of physician judgment, not law, and that brain death provided the right medical criterion—enjoyed support. When Curran wrote his Notes, a discernible legal literature pursued that goal.

LEGAL LITERATURE

Curran's Notes appeared at the end of at least a decade of writing in law review journals about whether physicians could transplant organs without being in violation of the law or vulnerable to suit. The tenuous legal position of transplantation—which according to critics was the reason physicians rushed into a definition of brain death—alarmed legal scholars. Soon after Joseph Murray completed the first human kidney transplant in 1954, a study in the *University of Detroit Law Journal* went in search of the legal basis that permitted a family member or any conscious individual to authorize the use of organs for transplant.[31] It found no such basis. Even so, by that time no instance of transplant had resulted in proceedings, in an American court, to charge a physician with battery, murder, or violation of rules regarding the handling of a corpse. Nor did any occur up to the final draft of the Uniform Anatomical Gift Act by the Commissioners on Uniform State Laws in July of 1968. Nonetheless, legal observers and advocates found that while the common law and statute could perhaps be read as providing justification for kin-approved or willed use of organs for transplant at the time of death, the legal basis for such authorization was not clear.

The *Detroit* paper mapped out an analysis and list of precedents that would be regularly referred to over the next decade in reviews of the legal environment for transplant. These included judicial rulings on the prerogatives of family members with respect to disposal of the body of a deceased person, limits on autopsy, and evolving statutes and case law regarding the ability of a person or family to permit use of the body for scientific purposes (usually for dissection and the teaching of anatomy). What emerged from these analyses was a claim to a somewhat uniquely American, common law, "quasi-property" interest that a family had in the dead body, thus granting family members some prerogative around its disposal, the means of which could also be established through a will. This diverged from British common law deference to ecclesiastical interest in the body that curtailed both testamentary prerogatives over the body and rights of the family. Legal scholarship during the following decade continued to highlight the ways in which the law was unprepared to regulate, let alone permit, transplantation. A perceived risk of criminal prosecution of transplant surgeons was attributed to laws such as those that prohibited unauthorized dissection of a corpse. Some lawyers searched the dense history of cases regarding the handling of corpses for a possible common law grounding that would allow people to will or instruct that upon death their body part(s) could be used for transplant or, similarly, to sanction next of kin to do likewise on their behalf.[32] The latter authorization had perhaps the least firm justification, as it was based in contested and complex rules about familial possession of the body.[33]

> With the exception of the few jurisdictions which have legislation concerning this problem [as of then, 1956, four states], the matter is one of the common law, which unfortunately affords no clear cut

answer to the legal effect of a donation of tissue...This nebulous area of the law needs clarification. The reasonable wishes of the deceased concerning the final disposition of his body should be paramount to all other interests...The same interest in medical and scientific progress which made possible the anatomical laws augurs social approval of the donation of one's body for the purposes of research or transplantation.[34]

Thus, in 1955 "it would seem fair to conclude that a person at the present time in the United States probably has the right to control the disposition of his body after death as long as no public policy is contravened, and it would seem to follow that an individual in his lifetime can give permission for the taking of tissue from his body after death."[35]

Commonly cited justifications for this conclusion in subsequent law review treatments of the topic rested on nineteenth-century adjudication of willed disposal of corpses; in particular, cases such as *Pettigrew v. Pettigrew* and *Pierce v. Swan Point Cemetery* reached back to the nineteenth century.[36] In the latter, it was argued that:

Although, as we have said, the body is not property in the usually recognized sense of the word, yet we may consider it as a sort of quasi property, to which certain persons may have rights, as they have duties to perform towards it arising out of our common humanity. But the person having charge of it cannot be considered as the owner of it in any sense whatever; he holds it only as a sacred trust for the benefit of all who may from family or friendship have an interest in it.

This case, and this particular section of it, was frequently cited as authority for extending numerous rights usually exercised over other property to include rights over a dead body. These rights included the ability to recover damages for mutilation and unauthorized disposal, or the authority to follow pre-decedent wishes regarding use.[37] But *Pierce* actually restricted the prerogatives of a surviving spouse over the corpse, as it emphasized the ways in which the corpse was a *quasi*-property, and thus recognized multiple claims at stake. Earlier in the opinion, the court described this "quasi property" right as the following:

> That there is no right of property in a dead body...may well be admitted...[However].... There is a duty imposed by the universal feelings of mankind to be discharged by some one towards the dead; a duty on the part of others to abstain from violation; it may therefore be considered as a sort of a quasi property.[38]

Specifically the court ruled here that a wife could not disinter her husband and relocate his remains against the daughter's wishes, as that seemed "improper conduct." The following one hundred years of jurisprudence in the United States regularly reexamined this tension between individual and community interest in the corpse and, over time, inched further toward regarding the corpse as an extension of the previously living person. Yet these cases seemed to provide particularly slim legal footing for families to secure the ability to give permission for organ removal for the purposes of transplant. The inference that legal difficulties would be avoided with familial consent—since such consent removed the only ones (i.e., family members of the deceased) with legal standing to challenge the procedure—was hardly firm ground.

The perception that case law was probably not hostile, but *was* still dangerously nonspecific with respect to lawful disposition of the body for transplantation purposes, persisted through the 1960s. Physicians became more concerned as increasing numbers of legal scholars wrote of these persistent gaps in the law. The CIBA Foundation–sponsored symposium on Ethics in Medical Progress in March of 1966 was an unprecedented gathering of individuals involved in transplantation worldwide, who met to discuss the legal and ethical aspects of the practice. It is, and was, often quoted for revealing how practices that resembled the brain death criteria were already followed in several medical centers in Europe. Its published deliberations appeared more preoccupied, though, with whether transplant was in fact legal in any jurisdiction, either in Europe or the United States. That doubt was primarily cast by existing law, not about death-defining, but about the disposition, dissection, and bequeathing of bodies.[39]

One active CIBA participant, law professor and surgeon Carl E. Wasmuth, continued to try to mine possible sources for a legal ability to transplant from common law and statute on burial and autopsies. Concluding that removal of organs for autopsy or scientific study required consent "by the person or persons who have the right of burial," it seemed logical to take the next step: "The right to remove organs for the purposes of transplantation into another person, therefore, depends upon the consent for the removal of such organs by the person who possesses the right of burial."[40] But even if this inductive leap would satisfy a judge, it was inadequate to the circumstances of transplantation. Actually relying on burial rights or medical examiner autopsy disposal prerogatives would involve decision making that was too slow for the time frame needed for removing tissues for transplant. While states passed statutes establishing methods for families and individuals to authorize tissue donation for the specific purpose of transplantation, by the time the Harvard Committee met the legal climate was still wanting, for reasons similar to those described in 1955. Alfred and Blair Sadler, who had been consultants in the effort by the National Conference of Commissioners on Uniform State Laws to draft the Uniform Anatomical Gift Act, reviewed much of the same legal precedent explored in the prior decade and found similarly that:

> The paucity of cases dealing with donation of tissue, by either the decedent or next of kin, and the conflicting judicial treatment of the questions dealing with the place and manner of burial, provide little assurance that an individual has the authority to control the disposition of his body.[41]

Similarly, autopsy statute interpretations did "not reveal a judicial willingness to extend the scope of autopsies by implication,"[42] and while some localities extended autopsy authorization to include removal of tissue for transplantation, as with corneas, this legal authority was impractical for tissues needed more immediately. The Sadlers reviewed the forty-one state statutes that, up to 1968, regulated tissue and organ use for transplant. They found that while many states finally granted explicit authority to families to permit tissue use for transplant, few fit the realities of whole-organ transplantation. These laws also varied so widely as to be impractical. The Uniform Anatomical Gift Act, which had just been endorsed by the American Bar Association, could, the Sadlers and others argued, address those deficiencies. But even that model legislation left open the question of when the deceased (from whose body the family could authorize use of organs) was, in fact, deceased. The Act vaguely left it to physicians to answer that question. Legal writers lingered on this issue more closely, though generally they too left the issue to physicians, generally endorsing some idea of brain death as described, and increasingly practiced, by several European physicians and by Robert Schwab.

Legal commentators closely examining potential and longstanding legal impediments to transplant generally acceded to medical authority over new criteria but also to the view that such a definition was hardly sufficient to address obstacles to transplantation that required the Uniform Anatomical Gift Act and other statutory changes to fill in where the common law on autopsies and cadavers had not. And as with concerns voiced by Curran and Beecher these links between brain death and transplant were also often made in order to *police* transplantation practice. The widely publicized case of kidneys retrieved from a brain-injured woman at the Karolinska Institute by Swedish surgeon Clarence Crafoord, for example, involved a patient with spontaneous breathing and circulation despite presumably irreparable loss of consciousness. Without clear medical consensus on stricter criteria, Wasmuth and others feared that dangerous unpredictability would reign in the use or abuse of medical technology, and they made reference to Nazi practices to underscore the point.

"We should distinguish," Keith Simpson, Professor of Forensic Medicine at Guy's Hospital in London, argued before the 1966 Fourth International Meeting of Forensic Medicine, "between being alive and a live state that can be maintained artificially...we can say that death has occurred if the brain is no longer in a living state, even if it can be maintained as living tissue by artificial means."[43] Despite assertions like this, the law as yet did not recognize this vocabulary of death before dying wherein "being alive" or in an "alive state," or being "no longer in a living state" but having "a living tissue" were key determinants.

Increasingly, however, other legal scholars advocated for this new sensibility and for physicians to standardize reliable criteria to bring the law more in line with this reality:

> With these illustrations, it becomes evident that death is no longer determined by the lack of respiration or the lack of a heartbeat or the lack of circulation. Death is determined by several factors but primarily by the state of unconsciousness. When the chances of recovery of consciousness have been totally eliminated, brain death has occurred...The question then is, "When is the brain so damaged that consciousness cannot be regained?" Medicine and the law then must define it upon medical principles that have been well established...The definition of death must fit within the modern concept of life as it is defined by the physiologist.[44]

This advocacy took place not only in the context of examining legal hurdles to transplantation but also in meeting broader reasons for a revised definition of death. As one law review article observed, a clear, revised definition of death was necessary for a variety of legal purposes, including assuring patients of the restraints that would be placed on physicians against unwarrantedly using their organs, and resolving legal ambiguities caused by the imprecision of the cardiopulmonary definition of death. It was heart-lung death that was too legally vague, imprecise, and thus dangerous. Pacemakers, cardiac resuscitation, and life support all created legal quagmires if cardiopulmonary death remained as the definition of death itself:

> If we continue to hold fast to the present legal definition of death as a cessation of perceptible heartbeat and respiration, in many instances

we can not only ask when a man died but how many times as well. The current definition presents many problems to both the legal and the medical world, for because of advances in medicine, it is no longer an event taking place at a precise time but rather is often a continuing event.[45]

Examining much of the same evidence as Curran, others drew less circumscribed conclusions than he did. Jeffrey C. Baker reviewed nearly all of the same simultaneous death cases, along with the 1963 Newcastle inquest, to conclude, as did the Committee, that the law would defer to physician criteria. But he went further, using these cases to show how awkward and problematic legal goals were—such as determination of the time or cause of death—in a world of life support, a world of death before dying. A revised legal understanding of death was needed to correct both "the disparity between medical and legal definitions of death" and to remedy the law's failure to address "the uncertainty that exists in present legal doctrine concerning the fact of death and when death occurs. In the absence of any case or statute in point, the law must then turn to medicine."[46] After reviewing medical evidence regarding the necessity of brain function for consciousness and autonomous life, along with the posited ability of EEG to assess brain activity, Baker concluded that "there is probably no malpractice liability if EEG recording time periods used are justified medically."[47] These features of medical practice, coupled with the limited guidance from case law, provided an argument for standardized consensus over new criteria for death. It was medicine's task to provide the details. Baker felt Schwab's criteria were conservative and actually a likely obstacle to transplantation. He mentioned other approaches—such as that of Peter C. Kellaway, Director of EEG at Houston's Methodist Hospital—which relied on EEG readings only. In contrast, Schwab, and eventually the Committee, required the absence of specific reflexes, responsiveness, and spontaneous respiratory activity.[48]

Starting over a decade before brain death appeared, then, a number of legal scholars had already described in similar ways the need for the law to catch up with changes in medical practices in terms of defining death. These predecessors also argued that brain death facilitated but did not solve the legal minefield that needed to be cleared for transplant while also providing other needed legal remedies. At a conference sponsored by Villanova University School of Law soon before the Report appeared, brain death was understood as a corrective so that the law could be more relevant to the challenges faced in hospitals. Clear consensus on the clinical description of brain death was needed to solve pressing problems above and beyond transplantation, such as the need to distinguish between ordinary and extraordinary treatment.[49]

Along these lines, George P. Fletcher, then on the law faculty at the University of Washington, published in 1967 a lengthy and widely quoted paper on the enduring issue of the differences between the omission, commission, and interruption of treatment. Even though no claims against a physician for removing respirator support had occurred up until then, it had been a common opinion that removal of treatment opened up physicians to charges of homicide.[50] Fletcher argued that turning off the respirator was not, in a legal-liability sense, a removal but an omission. He based this opinion "not so much on policy and analysis, as on acceptance of the received premises of the law of homicide."[51] Within the logic of homicide adjudication, such a removal of treatment by a physician would fall into the category of an omission rather than an act. This being established, the legal standard of defensible omissions would then hold sway in judging physician conduct. The standard was that in order to be legally permissible, the omitted behavior had to fall within the standard of care expected of a doctor toward a patient: "If it is an act, the relationship between the doctor and patient is [in the eyes of the law] irrelevant. If it is an omission, it is all controlling." This is where brain death came in. In this legal framework, brain death was a needed statement of professional care standards within which omissions were distinct from offensive, actively committed, acts: "The conclusion of our circular journey is that doctors are in a position to fashion their own law to deal with cases of prolongation of life. By establishing customary standards, they may determine the expectations of their patients and thus regulate the understanding and the relationship between doctor and patient."[52]

This was essentially the conclusion of the Committee itself. Legal journals and conferences in the years before the Report argued that brain death could close existing gaps in the law. It would appropriately and primarily address complications, presented by new technologies, that clouded consensus as to the limits and expectations of care for the seriously ill and that resonated within the familiar categories of omissions, commissions, and extraordinariness. It would not solve the legal impediments to transplant, for which Schwab's criteria were thought too narrow a response anyway. However representative this brief sampling of legal consensus of the time may be, it at a minimum captures the presence of a line of legal scholarly thinking about authority to redefine death and the ways in which this thinking was part of broader efforts around evidence-based standard-setting that mirrored the Committee's. Historical characterization of the Committee as an almost rogue operation of medical overreach needs to be revised, and the potential value of medical calculus and contexted knowledge reconsidered in historical context.

These examples also put into perspective later criticism of the Report for defining as "death" what could have simply been a good set of conditions for withdrawal of care. Such a position may not have had the maturity of acceptance and legal justification to qualify as a credible position to take at the time—even leaving aside the very different sorts of reasons that did lead Beecher, Schwab, and colleagues to see brain death as more than just a compelling cause for withdrawal but as death itself.

CASE LAW RESPONDS

The conclusions of the legal section of the Committee Report thus mirrored ongoing discussions in at least some parts of the legal literature, though not yet the case law that Curran cited. Courts and cases would soon follow that lead. Note, for example, a survivorship case appearing soon before the Report appeared. In a seemingly familiar narrative of possible simultaneous deaths, a couple in their second marriage—each with distinct heirs from their first—were found dead after a head-on car collision. A slumped and silent husband was compared to his unresponsive wife, who bled from her ears and in whom a bystander asserted he could feel a pulse, albeit one incompatible with survival as it was timed at five beats over one and a half minutes. Groans were audible, unclearly purposeful, and perhaps indicated the physical mechanics of demise. But other signs vied for relevance with these movements and sounds when a parade of experts juggled autopsy and witness observations:

> As indicated above, there was almost no conflict among all of the experts concerning the cause of Max's death and that he died almost instantaneously. As to Patricia, appellants' experts surmised that she also died instantaneously of an injury to her brainstem or a crushed spinal cord, basing their opinions on the condition of her pupils and the mediastinal hemorrhage. However, they admitted there was nothing in the testimony of the lay witnesses or the autopsy reports that was inconsistent with Patricia's survival and breathing for 10–20 minutes after the impact...Respondent's medical experts, basing their opinions chiefly on the uncontroverted heavy bleeding...surmised that Patricia did not suffer a brain stem severance or spinal cord injury, but died more slowly from a severe basal skull fracture.[53]

The court felt that the lower Superior Court's ruling in favor of the respondent was a reasonable one in light of the expert disagreement, but survivorship case law here includes inference and expanded literacy about brain function in its weighing of sufficiency of evidence for simultaneity—a legal viewpoint that would only grow.

Forward to 1987, when Cecil A. Hughes shot and killed his wife Suzanne Duperier Hughes and then turned the gun on himself with a fatal shot to the head. Suzanne was deemed to have lived longer based on the testimony of Suzanne's (not Cecil's) son. The son testified that after he found a motionless Cecil, Suzanne appeared to take some breaths for ten to twenty minutes after the shots. Because of this finding, their respective estates went to Suzanne and her heirs. Cecil's heirs challenged this finding in the Court of Appeals of Missouri. Much of the opinion reads like a 1950s survivorship case—indeed, many such cases are cited therein—with review of detailed testimony in the circuit court regarding who was breathing or bleeding. But the court paused as follows:

> One of the problems inherent in this case is that the development of medical technology has complicated the definition of that condition called "death." Many of the older precedents simply accepted the definition found in *Black's Law Dictionary*, i.e., "The cessation of life; the ceasing to exist; defined by physicians as a total stoppage of the circulation of the blood, and a cessation of the animal and vital functions consequent thereon, such as respiration, pulsation, etc." Nowadays, the development of "life-support systems" and the increasing use of human organ transplants have made the definition of "death" more complex.[54]

The appeal was denied, with the court finding it reasonable that the initial ruling not only found persistent life in Suzanne's movement but also that in Cecil's wound it found instant death through injury to the brain. Quickly, many courts started to sift through the minute details of brain death criteria, just as they had split hairs between gurglings and groans. In an example of how life can be tragically stranger than fiction, the Illinois Appellate Court heard an appeal of a simultaneous death ruling that involved spouses who collapsed together at home after taking Tylenol that was later discovered to have been laced with cyanide as part of a broader distribution of poisoned Tylenol that captured wide public attention at the time. The reason the couple sought pain relief was because they were distraught over the collapse and death that same day of the husband's brother—a death later found out to have been the result of exposure to the same tainted medication.

Wheeled into the emergency room, Stanley Janus died soon after his arrival there, as the presence of electrical heart activity could not be translated into effective heart movement and blood pressure, and he was declared dead some hours later. His wife Theresa never regained consciousness, and vying expert testimony disagreed as to whether she was brain dead at admission (she had no discernible heart activity on admission, but her heart was able to be revived and she was placed on a respirator) or two days later when death was specifically "declared." Expert witnesses disputed whether an EEG tracing showed "minimal electrical activity" or merely artifact in a portion of her brain, or whether one pupil briefly responded to light, as a nurse noted at 2:30 one morning.[55] While the court felt enough uncertainty to allow the finding that Theresa survived her husband, the world of whirring bodies was receding to one of neurological detail.

The narrow window for timing death as an event, and not a process—so crucial to the adjudication of simultaneity disputes and so central to the criticism and discomfort over Beecher's "arbitrariness"—opened up widely. Changes in the early 1990s to The Uniform Simultaneous Death Act departed from decades of adherence to an assumption of simultaneity simply in the absence of "contrary evidence" or "sufficient evidence." The suspended, prolonged parsing of death from dying was reflected in revisions requiring survival of 120 hours or more, as well as "clear and convincing evidence" of such survival in order to defy simultaneity.[56]

Post-Report survivorship cases departed from the blood and breathing concreteness of *Black's* upon which they had previously relied. According to a 1977 case:

> Moreover, although *Black's Law Dictionary* does not have the force
> of statute or even a judicial decision, we accept its definition of death
> as "cessation of life" or "ceasing to exist." But its assertion that death
> is defined by physicians in a certain way does not freeze the medical
> definition for all time, and its references to respiration and pulsation
> must be taken to refer to spontaneous rather than artificially
> supported functions.[57]

In 1960s legal literature, and in the assessment and legal advice of the Committee's distinguished scholar, legal barriers to transplantation were problems worth solving, but brain death was no panacea. Curran made clear the limited value of brain death to solving obstacles to transplant, and the Committee restricted its purview to where at least some early legal literature on this topic was urging it to go. From this medical-legal perspective, then, the Committee's work is hard to characterize as a back-door effort to make an experimental procedure normal, or to primarily advocate for transplant, let alone avoid legal scrutiny or protections over transplantation.

This background more interestingly opens up for consideration the degree to which brain death was aligned with a very different historical narrative: the use of medically derived knowledge and standards to sta-bilize legal frameworks. In the conversations and cross-talk between case law, physicians, and legal scholars, the *meanings* or *concepts* of death or duties that would later engage brain death critics seemed peripheral to the attention instead given to the contexts of the work and outcomes of medical care itself. The Committee was not alone in how it identified and predicted changes in case law, or in how it sought to close the gap between the experience of newer capabilities and older practices by making clear criteria for deciding when the brain was dead.

The neurological criteria themselves now get our attention. As with Beecher's justification, the Harvard definition emerged from a broader and deeper set of practices and historical developments than have generally been attributed to it. The story of the criteria similarly challenges assump-tions about the relative importance of ethical concepts—as opposed to complex medical facts themselves—as the key tools for describing values and establishing consensus over hard choices in medicine.

NOTES

1.   William Curran, "Some Notes on the Legal Meaning of Death," photocopy manu-script, Box 11, Folder 18, Beecher Papers.

2. M. Martin Halley and William Harvey, "On an interdisciplinary solution to the legal-medicine definitional dilemma in death," *Indiana Legal Forum* 2, no. 69 (1968): 219–37, 237.

3. Nikolas Rose, Joelle M. Abi-Rached, *Neuro: The new brain sciences and the management of the mind* (Princeton: Princeton University Press, 2013).

4. Ian A. Burney, *Bodies of Evidence: Medicine and the Politics of the English Inquest, 1830–1926* (Baltimore: Johns Hopkins University Press, 2000).

5. Curran, "Some Notes on the Legal Meaning of Death," 2. He specifically cited *Thomas v. Anderson* (96 Cal. App. 2d 371, 211 P. 2d, 478), and *Smith v. Smith* (229 Ark. 579, 317 S.W. 2d, 275), cases questioning the simultaneity versus sequential timing of deaths of family members in fatal accidents, and a British coroner's inquest in Newcastle in 1963. A good account of the latter case is in *Medicine, Science and Law* 4 (1964): 77. The inquest involved the question of whether a kidney donor was dead when his kidneys were removed.

6. Interviews with the author, Fred Plum, April 20, 1998; C. Miller Fisher, December 9, 1996. See also interview with Vincent Perlo, July 30, 1991, and MGH Medicine Chair. Perlo was a fellow of Fisher's and closely involved in the latter's efforts to establish an examination of the comatose patient useful in advising when to end treatment.

7. *Smith v. Smith*, 317 SW2d, 275, 276.

8. Curran, "Some Notes on the Legal Meaning of Death," 1. Curran is quoting from the Fourth Edition, 488.

9. Ad Hoc Committee, "A Definition of Irreversible Coma," 339.

10. Curran, "Some Notes on the Legal Meaning of Death," 8–9.

11. Curran to Beecher, May 8, 1968, Box 11, Folder 17, Beecher Papers.

12. Curran to Beecher, April 22, 1968, Box 11, Folder 24, Beecher Papers.

13. Ad Hoc Committee, "A Definition of Irreversible Coma," 339.

14. Sidney D. Rosoff and Robert S. Schwab, "The EEG in Establishing Brain Death. A 10-Year Report with Criteria and Legal Safeguards in 50 States," manuscript copy, Abstract, American Electroencephalographic Society presentation, Atlantic City, NJ, June 8, 1967. I am grateful to Dr. Schwab's surviving widow, Joan Schwab, for access to and permission to use this copy. This presentation is discussed further in Chapter Four.

15. Curran to Beecher, April 22, 1968, Beecher Papers, 2.

16. Ad Hoc Committee, "A Definition of Irreversible Coma," 339.

17. Ibid., 276.

18. Ibid., 277.

19. Ibid., 278.

20. J. F. Alderete, F. R. Jeri, E. P. Richardson Jr., S. Sament, R. S. Schwab, and R. R. Young, "Irreversible coma: A clinical electroencephalographic and neuropathological study," *Transactions of the American Neurological Association* 93 (1968): 16–20. See discussion of this paper in Chapter Five.

21. *Schmitt v. Pierce* 344 SW 2d, 120, 124.

22. Ibid., 125.

23. Ibid., 126–127.

24. Ibid., 133.

25. *Prudential Insurance Co. of America v. Spain*, 90 NE 2d, 256, 259, 258.

26. *Gray v. Sawyer*, 247 SW2d, 496. For similar reasoning privileging mechanical movement to brain function, see the 1938 case *Vaegermast v. Hess*, 280 NW, 641.

27. In re Di Bella's Estate, 199 Misc. 847, 100 NYS 2d, 763, 777.

28. *Taylor v. Cawood* 211 SW, 47, 51.

29. *Salingman's Estate* 13 Pa Dist. & Co. R. 2d, 432–34.

30. *Glover v. Davis*.

31. Allan D. Vestal, Rodman E. Taber and W. J. Shoemaker, "Medico-legal aspects of tissue homotransplantation," *University of Detroit Law Journal* 18, no. 3 (1955): 171–94.

32. Ibid., 185.

33. Again, much of the justification for this view was in nineteenth-century cases. See *Meagher v. Driscoll*, 99 Mass, 281 (1868); *Larsen v. Chase* 47 Minn, 307, 301, 50 NW, 238, 239 (1891).

34. Marvin I. Barish, "The law of testamentary disposition—A legal barrier to medical advance!", *Temple Law Quarterly* 30 (1956): 40–46, 45–46.

35. Vestal, Taber, and Shoemaker, "Medico-legal aspects of tissue homotransplantation," 187.

36. *Pettigrew v. Pettigrew*, 207 Pa 313, 56 Atl 878, 64 LRA 179 (1904) and *Pierce v. Swan Point Cemetery*, 10 RI 227 (1872).

37. In *O'Donnell v. Slack* 123 Calif. 285 (1899) it was declared: "It is recognized that the individual has a sufficient proprietary interest in his own body after his death to be able to make a valid and binding testamentary disposition of it." This was a case whereby a man expressed to his wife his wish to be buried in Ireland, where he was born. The estate administrator balked at funding such a trip for the body and his widow, but was ordered by a court to do so. For summaries of much of the case law behind finding pre-decedent disposal rights and the extent of the property right to care for a corpse, see the 1905 *Koerber v. Patek*, 102 NW 40 and the 1950 *Kirsey v. Jernigan* 17 ALR 2d 766.

38. *Pierce v. Swan Point Cemetery*, 238.

39. G. E. W. Wolstenholme and Maeve O'Connor, eds., *CIBA Foundation Symposium— Ethics in Medical Progress: With Special Reference to Transplantation* (Boston: Little, Brown, and Co., 1966).

40. Carl E. Wasmuth and Bruce H. Stewart, "Medical and legal aspects of human organ transplantation," *Cleveland-Marshall Law Review*, 442–71, 464.

41. Alfred M. Sadler Jr. and Blair L. Sadler, "Transplantation and the law: The need for organized sensitivity," *The Georgetown Law Journal* 57, no. 5 (1968): 5–54, 13.

42. Ibid., 14.

43. Quoted by Ayd in his manuscript "What is Death," 5, for the American Medical Association Second National Congress on Medical Ethics, Chicago, October 5, 1968, and in O. Ruth Russel, *Freedom to Die: Moral and Legal Aspects of Euthanasia* (New York: Human Sciences Press, 1975).

44. Wasmuth and Stewart, "Medical and legal aspects of human organ transplantation," 166.

45. Betty Wolf, "The need for a redefinition of death," *Chicago-Kent Law Review* 45, no. 2 (1968): 202–206, 203.

46. Jeffrey C. Baker, "Liability and the heart transplant," *Houston Law Review* 6 (1968): 85–112, 85, 91.

47. Ibid., 96.

48. Schwab also commented on how persistent brain death and life support for more than twenty-four hours significantly compromised organs for transplant. Yet, both the Report and Schwab recommended a minimum wait of twenty-four hours between serial EEGs.

49. "The medical, moral and legal implications of recent medical advances: A symposium," *Villanova Law Review* 13 (Summer 1968): 732–92.

50. See for example the remarks of Charles Orth, former Assistant State's Attorney: "The law states that if there is a duty to act, an omission to act is the same as a positive act…If there were a discontinuance of the efforts to prolong life on the part of the doctor, knowing that the discontinuance of thus effort would result in death, then he is guilty of murder in the first degree." Charles E. Orth Jr., "Symposium on Euthanasia," Medico-Legal Committee of the Medical and Chirurgical Faculty, the Bar Association of Baltimore City and the Maryland State Bar, *Maryland State MJ* 2 (March 1953): 120–40.

51. George P. Fletcher, "Prolonging life," *Washington Law Review* 42 (1967): 999–1016, 1012.

52. Ibid., 1015–16. For a similar argument see George P. Fletcher, "Legal aspects of the decision not to prolong life," *JAMA* 203, no. 1 (Jan. 1, 1968): 65–68.

53. "Estate of Max Schmidt," *67 Cal. Rptr. 847*, June 11, 1968, 853.

54. "In the Matter of the Estate of Cecil A. Hughes," *735 S.W. 2d 787* (1987), 790.

55. *Janus v. Tarasewicz, 482 N.E. 2d*, 418 (1985).

56. "Uniform Simultaneous Death Act," *Uniform Laws Annotated-Volume 8B Estate, Probate and Related Laws with Annotations from State and Federal Courts* (West Group, 2001): 147–58.

57. *Commonwealth v. Siegfried Golston, 366 NE 2d 744* (1977), 748.

4

The Criteria I: The Waking Brain and the Discourse of Consciousness

"Within the brain a central transactional core has been identified between the strictly sensory or motor systems of classical neurology...capable of grading the activity of most other parts of the brain."

—H. W. Magoun, *The Waking Brain, 1958*

"There are several ways for a body to be a body, several ways for consciousness to be consciousness."

—M. Merleau-Ponty, *Phenomenology of Perception, 1962*

How did some physicians come to describe the features of irreversible coma? Critics of the Committee asked what evidence supported the criteria and upon what basis the Committee arrived at the apparent assumption in the Report that meaningful consciousness was necessary for life. The evidence the Committee relied on included decades of clinical observations on coma and published reports on outcomes at Massachusetts General Hospital for patients with coma. Research on the neurology of consciousness also had an impact on the evolution of the criteria, but a complex one. This chapter and the one that follows look at these sources, focusing first on a background of research as to how the neurology of consciousness was understood.

There was a vibrant and largely forgotten research interest in the neurology of consciousness in the decades preceding the Report that cannot be fully described here. The approach, then, in this chapter is to outline the particular work on EEG and consciousness that several members of the Committee, primarily Schwab and Adams, specifically referenced and drew upon. It is almost as important to capture how much this work did *not* answer the questions Schwab and his colleagues faced, as to consider how much it did. Eventually this work—with all its ambiguities and limitations—helped answer two key questions: How accurately can the brain's activity, and especially signs of the irreversible loss of activity, be "seen"? What are the consequences of these visible signs for drawing conclusions about the functioning of consciousness *and* of the body?

ELECTRICOCENTRIC LIFE

By the summer of 1967, Schwab estimated that he had consulted on approximately 150 cases in which a simple set of criteria that he had developed were used to end treatment. The connection between the demise of the brain and death had interested Schwab since the beginning of his MGH career. In 1941, in cooperation with the Boston Medical Examiner William Brickley, he performed a continuous EEG and EKG tracing on a patient in the MGH emergency ward who had a fatal spinal cord injury and "would surely die in a few hours." There was no respirator used to treat a patient with such an injury at the time. The two men were brought together out of a mutual interest in the question of which electrical activity persisted longer, heart or brain, and the subsequent question of what role EEG could have in determining time of death. Schwab's description of the event continued:

> Five minutes before death the right side showed no electrical activity
> at all but there was a single burst of rather normal appearing alpha

activity on the left side. Respiration ceased at 6:44 as is shown by movement artifact produced by the doctor placing the stethoscope on the chest. The amplitude of the electrocardiogram became very low. Although there was no pulse discernible the amplifier recorded the electrocardiogram when the amplitude was raised…There was no electroencephalographic recording from this point on. All electrical activity ceased…eight minutes after death but the heart resumed spontaneous activity one minute later. Twenty-six minutes after death moving the chest produced three abnormal electrocardiographic beats. There was nothing in the electroencephalogram…It is obvious from this example that the electrocardiogram is a better indicator [of the exact time of death].[1]

Thirteen years later, Schwab was confronted with another case:

[I was] called to the hospital on an emergency Saturday evening where a patient about to be operated on for a large intracranial clot had stopped breathing, was immediately put on a respirator, and maintained with normal heart, blood pressure. There was no visible sign of response to stimuli. Reflexes were totally absent, and the question arose as to what to do with the operating room about to close for the night and Sunday. The electroencephalogram was recorded…and there was nothing whatever to see in the tracing. The question was, "Is this patient alive or dead?" Without reflexes, without breathing, and with a total absence of evidence of an electroencephalogram, we considered that this patient was dead in spite of the presence of an active heart maintaining peripheral circulation. The respiration was therefore turned off and the patient pronounced dead.[2]

The latter description is presumably the first known description of the use of a brain death construct to determine death in the history of medicine. It is dramatic to compare these two deaths. They describe two fundamentally different conclusions drawn by Schwab as to criteria for determination of death—absent heart activity in the first; absent EEG tracing, reflexes, and breathing in the second. But in the 1941 impromptu experiment, death was defined only in part by the heart stopping. The degree to which the action of the heart as a pump drew the line between life and death was undermined by finding that electricity outlived the pulse. The electricity of the body, specifically of the heart, persisted beyond any value of the heart as a mechanically effective pump.

Through this electrical window, the body looked different. Schwab gives no indication in his account that he thought of using EEG to define death when he followed the tracing with Brickley. However, a quarter of a century later he listed this event at the start of a chronology of events leading to his criteria for brain death, which he prepared for an anticipated manuscript with Curran on "cerebral death" soon after the Report appeared.[3] Schwab ranked this vigil with Brickley second in importance only to 1930s physiological research that demonstrated permanent loss of EEG in experimental animals after the interruption of circulation to the brain. Yet his publications before the late 1950s—including a review, which also appeared in 1941, of the varying uses of EEG—made no mention of the possible role of EEG in determining death or even prognosticating cerebral function after anoxic injury.[4] Schwab's description of the Brickley episode was not presented to a larger clinical audience until a decade later in his textbook on EEG. It was described there in order to simply demonstrate the relative persistence of different electrical currents in the body, not as an observation in support of reconsidering the physiological markers used for determining death.[5] As Schwab later wrote, "Dr. Brickley was seeking information as to how long the brain survived after the heart ceased to beat."[6] In fact, his account first appeared in a forum unlikely to reach the attention of any physician: the pages of *Electrical Engineering*, in 1941. Here, observations of this dying patient appeared as a footnote to a published excerpt of the EEG tracing itself, presented again to illustrate the variable persistence of electrical currents in different tissues. Basic physiologic properties of tissues, not new methods of prognostication and definition, were the focus.

But we can glimpse with Schwab the newly layered confusions of past and present tenses in the definition of life that this new way of seeing the body, this new structuring of knowledge, brought:

> Brain waves disappear ten minutes before death. Legal death [occurred]....when intern placed stethoscope on chest to prove inaudible heartbeat...Electrocardiogram continues one minute after death, stops and then begins again.[7]

Forward to 1954, when everything seems to have changed compared with the 1941 case, *despite* persistent heartbeat, death was found because of loss of brain electricity and physical signs of brain functioning. In 1954, that persistence lost the significance it previously had. There are three ideas, though, that unite these two accounts even in their differences. First is an "electricocentric" account of biology: that electrical cellular activity either could replace or more precisely reveal functional attributes of an organ and/or the organism—attributes critical to the reliable determination of it as living. Second is the suspicion that loss of brain electrical activity was the final event of human life. Third, and more implicit, is the emerging understanding that death was a slippery construct without clear lines or technical or clinical signs. Death did not close a door on an array of other continuing biological events that were a part of dying.

Other key changes between 1941 and 1954 included the use of respirators as well as the growth of EEG-based research in describing consciousness and brain function. This chapter describes a largely forgotten burst of EEG studies in the mid-twentieth century, focusing specifically on how they framed Schwab's purposes on the wards of MGH where respirator-dependent patients elevated the visibility and relevance of electricocentric life.

This research changed how physicians talked about patients, such as a man, age nineteen, who suffered the end-stage results of a growing brain tumor. Hospitalized in Britain, the patient was cared for by British neurologist Kinnier Wilson, early in his career. Wilson later wrote:

> June 23, 1905, at 11.10 pm, I was called to see the patient. He was lying on his back, with head turned slightly to the right, and was

quite unconscious... When the lids were lifted the eyes were seen to be fixed and staring straight front... 11.45 p.m. About this time both arms became rigid, the left elbow rather more than the right... This striking position of the arms was henceforth maintained; at intervals the whole arm would stiffen still further, as it were, and the attitude become more accentuated, as if by waves of contraction passing down the musculature... 12.20 a.m. Another fit started. Patient suddenly became absolutely stiff in the decerebrate position, and his face reddened, while respiration became occasionally labored, down to four per minute... The eyes were open, staring straight in front; pupils were dilated to their widest and did not react to light... The phenomena exhibited by the patient during these hours resemble in minute particulars those of mesencephalic transection in experimental animals. Until hemorrhage and increasing pressure killed him he was little more than a decerebrate preparation.[8]

The author considered this man's condition and those of similar patients to be analogous to a "decerebrate preparation" used in experiments with animals. These kinds of experiments were developed by Charles Sherrington, who was awarded the 1932 Nobel Prize in Medicine for his work on the basic architecture of nerve cells as fundamental units of brain function.[9] In the experiments, the area between the cerebral hemispheres and upper spinal cord was severed. Higher cuts, up closer towards the brain hemispheres and cortex, such as in the midbrain, produced the typical rigid, deformed, or "decerebrate" responses that Wilson described. Lower cuts, moving in the opposite direction toward the spinal cord and into the brainstem, caused flaccid unresponsiveness instead.

Tumors or bleeding in this same region, or pressure exerted on this region by similar lesions in other parts of the brain that expanded in the closed space of the skull, created unfortunate human equivalents of these laboratory models, with varying abnormalities in breathing and in reflexes of the cranial nerves (i.e., reflexes of central nervous system nerves within the skull such as pupil, cornea, and other eye movements and reflexes). The anatomy of the nuclei, or centers, of cranial nerves was well understood in this part of the nervous system, and it had been known since the turn of the nineteenth century that destruction of a certain part of the lower brainstem ended respiration. Tracking cranial nerve and limb movements became the basis of a neurological examination that used external signs to locate injury in the cortex and lower brain regions such as the brainstem. What changed over time was the explanation of what these signs meant, and especially what they meant for the machinery of consciousness and the overall prognosis for survival.

The association between irreversible brain injury and loss of circulation or adequate oxygenation was also quite old. Humane societies in the eighteenth century were well aware of the need to rapidly resume halted breathing lest it reach a point beyond which resuscitation was impossible.[10] Study of the effects of anoxia on nerve cells and nervous system function is almost two hundred years old. Twentieth-century research often cited Astley Cooper's 1836 publication on arterial occlusion in rabbits.[11] At the turn of the twentieth century, a fairly hefty scientific literature existed exploring the histological changes that occurred in nerve cells when deprived of oxygen. These studies were meant to answer the still vexing question of what aspects of anoxic injury to cells indicated "which of them might recover under proper conditions, and which of them were injured beyond the possibility of recovery."[12]

In 1934, with EEG technology (and agreement that it in fact reflected activity in the brain) less than a decade old, Simpson and Derbyshire reported in the *American Journal of Physiology* that disappearance of detectable electrical activity occurred within approximately twenty seconds of experimentally produced anoxia in the cat motor cortex.[13] Experiments by Sugar and Gerard, frequently cited by Schwab, demonstrated how areas of the brain lost discernible EEG when deprived of oxygen at different rates.[14] So, while neatly linked together, the leap from positing a physiological relationship between cell death and loss of EEG to (eventually) a complete map of irreversible loss of specific brain functions, was a work in progress.

TURNING CONSCIOUSNESS ON ITS HEAD: THE WAKING BRAIN VERSUS THE AFFERENT BRAIN

During the mid-1930s, experiments by Belgian researcher Frederic Bremer found that cats with severed, or transected, midbrains had EEG patterns similar to those seen during sleep. This level of brain isolation, called *cerveau isole*, was contrasted with transection lower down in the brainstem, which resulted in isolation of the whole brain, or *encephale isole*. The encephale cats showed wakefulness and nonsleep EEG patterns. These cat brains were still able to receive afferent—or incoming—sensory signals from the rest of the nervous system. The higher transection, cerveau isole, cut off more of these afferent connections. The prevailing deafferentation hypothesis—that alertness and consciousness were fueled by activation from afferent sensory information received from the body—thus seemed confirmed by these experiments.

These findings were soon linked to an earlier focus of EEG research—the so-called Berger Rhythm. EEG research initially studied single nerve potentials, the speed of nerve signal transmission, and paths of transmission in different parts of the nervous system. This kind of study portrayed an electrical brain characterized by momentary, local, and rapidly changing electrical bursts from one point to another. Berger, however, in the late 1920s and early 1930s, described a stable, persistent, generalized, and "slow" electrical rhythm that usually appeared on EEG at rest with closed eyes. When eyes opened or attention focused, the rhythm disappeared. The presence of a stable electrical rhythm in the human brain was not immediately accepted. However, Edgar Adrian and Bryan H. C. Matthews—established researchers in nervous system electrical potentials—confirmed and thus legitimated Berger's findings in 1934. Adrian had just shared the Nobel Prize with Sherrington. He and Matthews offered evidence that the rhythm reflected the electrical characteristics of the brain, particularly the occipital area, when at rest.[15] Some controversy persisted as to how much of the brain could produce this rhythm,[16] but what emerged was an enormously influential model of electrical brain activity, which showed that there were stable, predictable patterns of electrical waveforms associated with different overall states of the brain such as attention, concentration, sleep, or rest. In general, research about consciousness and emotion shifted from studying people and their reported reactions and emotions to something known and observed through brain activity. EEG was an important part of that shift.[17]

Berger's effort to measure brain electricity was part of a search for tangible signs of what he referred to as psychic energy, or "P. E." P. E. was the physical, measurable aspect of thought and experience, the product of a series of energy transformations ultimately originating in God.[18] These spiritual and holistic commitments were at odds with an emphasis by many contemporaries on unique, specialized functions of localized parts of the brain, as well as with later cybernetic, machine-mechanism metaphors for explaining consciousness, which proliferated in the 1950s and were strengthened through EEG-based research. These meanderings through localized, holistic, mechanical, and ephemeral metaphors for consciousness would continue over the following decades and produce a rich range of theories and experimental programs.[19] It is worth revisiting that range in order to later contrast the degree to which similar metaphorical and conceptual descriptions were used in the critical bioethics literature in the decades following the Report, to argue over what type of loss of consciousness was—or should be—at stake in defining brain death and personhood. Used for that purpose, however, these descriptions of how the brain worked were generally stretched beyond their concrete referents of events in the brain such that they became consequentially detached from a process of medical knowledge-making.

Berger's rhythm consisted of "synchronized," regular, low-voltage waveforms that occurred during states such as sleep and relaxation and that could be disrupted and replaced by high-voltage, erratic, or "desynchronized" patterns with accompanying arousal, alertness, and focused attention. Producing desynchronization—that is, provoking and observing this shift away from an intrinsic, synchronized, electrical pattern—became a common experimental procedure. Desynchronization could be shown in cats with an encephale isole condition—transection at the first cervical vertebrae that spared cranial nerve connections and thus maintained significant sensory input to the brain. But in cerveau isole cats, in which these connections were severed, neither arousal (as evidenced in behavior or EEG pattern) nor desynchronization of the sleep EEG could be produced. Disruption from somnolence to alert behavior, and the accompanying desynchronization of EEG, occurred in encephale cats and not cerveau cats. This was interpreted by Bremer to show that arousal relied upon afferent stimulation through the usual pathways of sensory information from the body that converged in the brain. The loss of sensory afferents, or deafferentation, turned the brain "off."

Others began to doubt that picture, considering instead that these transections were cutting into a lower brain center that wasn't just a passage way for afferent traffic but a control center that manipulated these alternating electrical patterns of arousal and somnolence, synchronization and desynchronization—essentially acting as an electrical pacemaker of the functioning brain. According to this understanding, the lower brain areas were not merely passive cables that conveyed afferent stimulation that would, if severed, shut down the cortex. These lower areas instead actively managed this activity.

Research on the mechanism of sleep similarly suggested the possibility of active centers of consciousness. The American neuroanatomist Stephen Ranson, who directed the Institute of Neurology at Northwestern University for over forty years, attributed somnolence caused by certain hypothalamic lesions in monkeys to be due to the lesions' impairment of the excitatory signals of that region. Withdrawal of those signals presumably caused sleep. Arousal, then, perhaps resulted from an intrinsic sophisticated electrical generator in midbrain or lower brain structures rather than from passive conveyance of sensations from the body. These structures actively caused *waking*, not sleeping. But this meant the lower centers did more than merely throw the switch for deafferentation. They selectively initiated and maintained arousal and consciousness directly. Electrophysiological study of these centers also expanded the ability to appreciate, distinguish, and argue about, the differences between these often non-distinguished terms ("arousal," "alertness," "consciousness,").

In a seminal 1949 paper, Guiseppi Moruzzi and Horace W. Magoun provided evidence that bolstered this view of the active role of these centers, and accelerated new ways of thinking about consciousness.[20] Stimulation of the "reticular activating system," or RAS (a particular area of interconnecting fibers coursing through the brainstem) caused desynchronization even when other sensory nerves to the brain were cut.[21] Transections of RAS blocked desynchronization. A complementary study was led by Donald Lindsley, a colleague at Northwestern University. Lindsley made important contributions to diverse fields such as learning, sleep, the behavior of animals in the wild, and challenges of long-term space flight. He joined Magoun in the latter 1950s to help create the Brain Research Institute at UCLA. When Lindsley and his research team destroyed RAS in "mesencephalic or diencephalic lesions...EEG activation was reduced or abolished and recurrent spindle bursts, like those of normal sleep or barbiturate anesthesia, dominated the cortical record."[22] From this he concluded:

> The evidence given above points to the presence in the brain stem of a system of ascending reticular relays, whose direct stimulation activates or desynchronizes the EEG, replacing high-voltage slow waves with low-voltage fast activity. This effect is exerted generally upon the cortex and is mediated, in part, at least, by the diffuse thalamic projection system.[23]

EEG provided the opportunity to distinguish not only anatomical but functional relationships between areas of the brain. This line of experimentation involved a who's who of twentieth-century neurophysiology, such as Nobel Laureate Walter Rudolph Hess, Ranson (who also taught Magoun in his doctoral thesis work), Robert Morison, Edward Dempsey, and Herbert Jasper. Jasper collaborated with the celebrated neurosurgeon Wilder Penfield, who did influential work in redescribing the nature of consciousness through brain stimulation of patients awake during surgery for epilepsy.[24]

The interaction between cortical and subcortical systems was a central focus of their work. Dancing and responding waveforms offered a new vision of the living brain. These waveforms not only made brain activity ostensibly visible; in this guise, they revealed brain function as orchestrated arousals emanating from small areas deep below the cortex. Speaking at a conference in Magoun's presence, Jasper presented a paper that concluded:

> The evidence to be brought forward by Magoun and his colleagues is in support of the relationship to spontaneous cerebral activity to the reticular portion of the brainstem independent of the main specific afferent pathways. The more diffusely interconnected, but topographically organized thalamic reticular system…provides a central coordinating mechanism for cerebral activities.[25]

The EEG vastly enlarged the available vocabulary with which to coherently claim that core functions of the brain and the phenomena of consciousness could be found below the cerebral hemispheres. This interest in the brainstem as the source of consciousness preceded the EEG. Within twentieth-century neurology literature, it was often traced to the kind of turn-of-the-century physiology captured in Martin Reichardt's 1908 argument that the brainstem contained an almost mystical vegetative engine, the "Antrieb," which provided the impetus, momentum, or source for life. The cortex permitted awareness of this impetus, and its capacity for reason balanced the Antrieb's momentum to create a harmonious organism.[26] Experience with patients further reinforced attention below the cortex in disturbances of consciousness in decorticate patients like Wilson's and the 1920s experience with epidemics of *encephalitis lethargica,* a disease characterized by a prolonged "sleep." Constantin von Economo, who characterized this frightening illness, associated its sleep or coma with damage just above the midbrain. This seemed consistent with previously known associations between other "vegetative" functions, such as body temperature and respiration, and similar areas of the brain.

In the 1930s, EEG tracings of slow, synchronized waveforms were obtained in patients with hypothalamic tumors, a human cerveau isole.[27] Lindsley made the connection between the desynchronization role of RAS and "the clinical observation of somnolence following basal injury to the brain."[28] The interpretation of loss of consciousness as the result of a damaged lower brain center that maintained it increasingly challenged the prevailing understanding of a cortical/subcortical division of labor. The latter view, more common at the time, was well summarized in a popularized account of neuroscience in the 1920s and 1930s by University of Chicago scientist C. Judson Herrick:

> The thalamus supplies the emotional coloring...the simple impulsive drives; the cortex supplies the intelligence guidance and rational control. The cerebral cortex at the top of the nervous axis is the center of highest dominance, and it exerts more or less control over all the lower centers and through these over everything the body does.[29]

Herrick's popularized physiology was, however, itself a critical response to the so-called James-Lange theory of emotion, attributed to William James and C. G. Lange. They independently argued that emotion was, as James put it, "the feeling of the bodily changes as they occur."[30] Herrick reestablished the cortex as more the driver than the recipient of emotions, but also acknowledged the need to break down the division of labor between local brain regions, attributing machine-like mechanisms to the brain. Machines, Herrick argued, were not dry or dehumanized entities. Instead, like the body and brain, machines moved energy for specific purposes. Unlike Berger, Herrick was opposed to spiritualist and holistic agendas, but still found it hard to talk about the brain without a teleological bent. EEG was also used by Hess to argue for a larger vision—in this case, that the harmonization of vegetative and animal energies it portrayed could be a roadmap for peaceful societies.[31] Appeals to holism in science have served many purposes over time,[32] and EEG provided an empirical basis for both mechanistic and holistic visions to reject a mind–body dualism.

EEG-based research on arousal and consciousness, then, fueled vying agendas and paradigms for the life sciences—a profusion of metaphors and models that were often contradictory. Commitments to holism, localization, mechanism, dualism, or higher agency were all projected onto bits of evidence about how consciousness worked.

In many ways this terrain did not much differ from the back and forth over the proper way to conceptualize life, identity, mind, and consciousness, in the ethical debates that later swirled around brain death, and that will be revisited in Chapter Six. In sharp distinction from much of that later debate, this earlier round of conceptual and metaphysical categories was instructively different in terms of the degree to which such discourse related to medical and neuroscientific domains. These conceptual schema were sorted and arbitrated as they linked with and matched up against experiment and, especially in Schwab's case, clinical experience. What was useful for care emerged from that process. The EEG was a crucial translator for that linkage and iterative learning.

THE EXPERIENCE OF RAS-CYBERNETICS, PHENOMENOLOGY, AND THE DYNAMIC "I"

The possibilities presented by this new description of a dynamic brain were evident in a 1953 UNESCO symposium that brought together the key investigators—Adrian, Bremer, Hess, Jasper, Magoun, Moruzzi, Morison, and Penfield among them. That group also included Mary Brazier of MGH, a member of both Beecher's Department of Anesthesiology and a collaborator with Schwab's research team. Magoun recalled the event as an anxious coming of age of his work—an opportunity for legitimacy as well as new criticism.[33]

Old vocabularies took on new meanings to describe consciousness. "Integration" in particular became a common—though complex—metaphor. In the nineteenth century, British neurologist Hughlings Jackson found integration in layered functions of the "lower" nervous system, but still posited the frontal lobes of the cortex as the high seat of consciousness. However, integration in the hands of many RAS researchers upended this schema. When Wilder Penfield selectively applied small electrical shocks to the exposed brains of his conscious patients in the 1930s, he was struck by how observed muscle movements or experiences reported by the patient could occur, but be understood by the subject as either not real or not of their own purposeful making. The persistence of an experienced "I" that was sustained through this electrical hijacking of the cortex led Penfield to conclude:

> [I]t seems reasonable to assume that there is a discrete area of the brain the integrity of which is essential to the existence of conscious activity...a level of integration much higher than that to be found in the cerebral cortex, evidence of a regional localization of the neuronal mechanism involved in this integration...[lying] not in the new brain but the old.[34]

Penfield tweaked familiar words and a more familiar, Jacksonian heritage of progressive, ordered, sensorimotor "integrations" but turned these terms literally on their heads.

This view of consciousness faced many challenges, not only within neurology but elsewhere in the biological and social sciences. Listen, for example, to the five-year conversation between various leading figures in American science, sociology, anthropology, and psychiatry sponsored by the Macy Foundation.[35] Annually from 1950 to 1954, the foundation gathered notable behavioral scientists such as NIMH Director Seymour S. Kety, Talcott Parsons, Margaret Mead, and prominent psychiatrists. Donald Lindsley was also included, as was Henry Beecher.[36]

This Macy-sponsored conversation contained a rich palette of themes, investigatory strategies, and metaphors used to describe consciousness. Psychoanalytic descriptions of personality formation shared the meeting agenda with reviews of how glucose was used by the brain. Some argued for limiting the study of consciousness to measurable behaviors; others felt consciousness essentially was not an isolatable object of study but an introspective, subjective experience. In a telling statement, one participant, reflecting on the five-year experience, summarized well my own impression of the transcripts in terms of where the group stood: "So, although I still do not know what anybody else means when he says 'consciousness,' I have a much better understanding as to what I mean by it, even though I cannot put it into words."[37]

Lindlsey presented the desynchronization/RAS findings of Moruzzi and Magoun, and the use of EEG at times seemed to anchor the group's conversation, proving versatile enough to serve very different approaches to consciousness. It could incorporate psychoanalytic and sociological paradigms whereby RAS served as an intermediary, rendering the "symbolization" of stimuli at the heart of consciousness as well as satisfying a shared objective to more concretely measure and objectify research in this area. Nonetheless, the Conference ended without a dominant, shared narrative. While the methodological rigor and flexible application of EEG were useful for incorporating a range of paradigms, EEG research on subcortical activity and consciousness did not make its case across this audience. As one program presenter wrote, "I think the arguments that Penfield, Jasper and some of the others make about subcortical centers are beside the point, because an isolated cortex is useless to an animal."[38] Whether or not that was so—in what ways lower functions were necessary as opposed to sufficient for consciousness, and for physiologic survival—became a central question for Schwab's and others' efforts to treat and examine coma.

THE INTERESTS OF THE CLINIC

The claims put forth by Moruzzi, Magoun, Jasper, Morison, Lindsley, and a growing roster of investigators did, however, resonate with many other audiences. For Stanley Cobb, the founding Chief of Psychiatry at MGH, EEG could advance understanding of his own point of view that consciousness was "a function of nervous tissue in action, just as much as contraction is a function of muscle... What is needed is a method that will quantitatively determine the amount of some physiochemical process that parallels what we know about consciousness."[39]

At a "symposium on the brain and the mind" that took place at the annual meeting of the American Neurological Association in June of 1951, Magoun, Penfield, and Jasper made such claims explicit and further argued that their work could fill the need for such a method. Responded one participant at that event:

The suggestions of Dr. Magoun and Dr. Jasper and their co-workers that the lower brainstem levels exercise an important influence over the conditions of awareness and responsiveness are fascinating and open up great fields for further investigation by means of methods which have not hitherto been available.[40]

Cobb was among a network of medical investigators whom the Rockefeller Foundation, especially through the initiatives of Alan Gregg, turned to in an effort to unravel the connections between brain and mind. Cobb saw RAS and EEG research as an opportunity to break from the dominant hold of the cortex and consider new models more amenable to experimental study. Linking the complexity of a mass of neurons with the phenomenon of consciousness required breaking a code. Biological systems can often be reduced to recombinations of basic patterns of protein function or chemical reactions that can be manipulated and amplified to do many things, much the way that all of language relies on a few sounds or letters. What then, Cobb asked, were the basic elements, or letters, of consciousness?

The increasing focus on RAS-consciousness connections, along with a patterned-building-blocks approach to the biology of consciousness, led to other possibilities for understanding EEG signals. Instead of reflecting some general working state of the whole brain, perhaps the Berger rhythm and others were each one of a core set of possible brain states. Through desynchronization, RAS selectively manipulated these states in versatile sequences or combinations, like playing many melodies from a few keys or notes, so as to queue selected attention for the cortex. This possibility explained certain experimental phenomena that were otherwise difficult to account for. For example, beta rhythms over motor cortex desynchronized only immediately before the initiation of the act of clenching a fist, then quickly returned to baseline soon after the initiation despite the persistence of the observable clenching action.[41] Rather than marking conscious activity itself, perhaps desynchronization was part of a mechanism that recruited cells to implement the work of types of conscious activity.

RAS experiments could suggest that the reticulum helped order and manage where the cortex should place its attention. The basal rhythm of the brain, in this scenario, was then misleading if understood directly as the unity of active conscious activity. Adrian, who helped established Berger's rhythm as real, came to see it in this way—as the appearance of what the brain does when *not* participating in consciousness. The basal rhythm was a holding pattern. Desynchronization, then, would be the key event of full consciousness. It provided a mechanism for selectively directing the attention of certain neuronal networks and making them specifically accessible to the messages that reached them. The brain needed a centralized relay, parceling out cortical freedom from the alpha rhythm to be briefly and specifically engaged with (and of use to) the body.[42]

That orchestration of moment-to-moment changes in patterns of desynchronization, though, seemed at odds with the continuous and free-floating experience of consciousness. But perhaps that continuous experience was misleading and was different than the biological reality underlying it. French neuroscientist Alfred Fessard argued that "one can be conscious without being conscious of one's self." The continuous "I" sense of consciousness could be an artifact. In yet another twist on the metaphor of "integration," Fessard suggested that experienced integration, or "EI," was the core phenomenon of our experience and that "the essentiality of EI can be assumed to be present in the most primitive forms of sensibility as well as the highest levels of intellectual life."[43] "Integration" by the brain of the sequence of events comprising thought made consciousness seem unified when it was in fact built from fragmentation, from a constantly edited set of rapidly sequenced snapshots. As Cobb put it, "mind is the integration itself."[44] RAS was the integrator.

The idea of achieving unrestricted effects by varying the sequence and pattern of a restricted set of neuron patterns—Cobb's "letters of the alphabet"—made it plausible, to some, for a limited menu of properties in a functional center like RAS to be able to mediate diverse behavioral outputs. This concept had a strong and mutually reinforcing connection to the explosive field of "cybernetics" exemplified in Norbert Weiner's 1948 publication of *Cybernetics: or Control and Communication in the Animal and the Machine.*[45] The connection was explicitly made in books, papers, and transcribed conference discussions. At the 1951 American Neurological

Association meeting, Cobb cited MGH's Mary Brazier's observation that work by Weiner and the field of cybernetics resulted in a "change in concepts of the nervous system...so great that it is almost impossible to overestimate it. In brief, it is a change from the concept of a passive, static nervous system, to an active, dynamic one."[46] Weiner summarized much of that impact:

> I was compelled to regard the nervous system in much the same light as a computing machine, and I communicated this idea to my friend Rosenbleuth and to other neurophysiologists. I managed to get a group...together at Princeton for an informal session, and I found on the part of each group a great willingness to learn what the other groups were doing to make use of their terminology. The result was that very shortly we found that people working in all these fields were beginning to talk the same language, with a vocabulary containing expressions from the communication engineer, the servomechanism man, the computing-machine man, and the neurophysiologist. For example, all of them were interested in the storage of information to be used later, and all of them found that the word *memory*...was a convenient term to cover the whole scope of these different fields. All of them found that the term *feedback*, which had come from the electronics engineer...was an appropriate way of describing phenomena in the living organism as well as in the machine. All of them found that it was convenient to measure information in terms of numbers of yeses or noes, and sooner or later they decided to term this unit of information the *bit*. This meeting I may consider the birthplace of the new science of cybernetics, or the theory of communication and control in the machine and the living organism.[47]

Warren S. McCullough emphasized this focus on the on-off property of neuro-information:

> When an impulse reaches the end of a nerve fiber, it combines with various other impulses that have reached the same level to determine

whether the next nerve fiber discharges. In other words...the nerve fiber is a logical machine in which a later decision is made on the basis of the outcome of a number of earlier decisions. This is essentially the mode of operation of an element in a computing machine.[48]

For these investigators, the objects of the study of mind shifted from cells, membranes, and anatomy to the characteristics of the movement of on-off information, the behavior of binary systems of communication and computation, and the reconfiguration of "representations of life and society as systems of decisions and signals." Taken together, "it was a techno-epistemic transformation."[49]

Cybernetics also proved quite an elastic umbrella. It supported the idea of a small, defined, neuronal switching station as key to consciousness. Weiner used Lindsley's findings of a subcortical gating mechanism to justify his own views of the alpha EEG rhythm as a kind of clock that regulated neuroreactivity.[50] At the same time this viewpoint was aligned with a different, more spatially and functionally diffuse description of brain activity. Lashley, for example, was critical of work on RAS and yet his experiments were also a resource to cybernetic investigators interested in the brain.[51] Lashley's research in the 1920s addressed the seemingly endless dispute over localization versus diffusion of cortical functions. Since at least the nineteenth century, experiments that removed chunks of animal cortex found, in many cases, few significant effects. Lashley quantified removal and its impact on standardized problem-solving tasks by rodents, such as navigating a maze path and then recalling it in later trials. He found that only the amount of tissue destroyed, not the particular region, interfered with learning and recall. This research was itself pursued in response to prevailing theories of the time in which the accumulation and reinforcement of local and specific neuronal reflex arcs mediated thinking. Instead, Lashley offered a vision of dispersed cortical neuronal capacity for those functions:

Such facts can only be interpreted as indicating the existence of some dynamic function of the cortex which is not differentiated with respect to single capacities....In this there is close harmony with theories of a general factor determining efficiency in a variety of activities.[52]

Lashley argued that neural cortical material had, as a core property, "reso-nances," and, further that predictable, quantifiable rules governed such neuronal "resonators" to manage and "integrate" the activity of the brain. A basic set of resonator properties, dispersed throughout the pluripoten-tial cerebral cortex, rather than highly localized and specific functions, made the brain work.

Revisiting these diverse (and vying) mechanistic and holistic, local and diffuse characterizations of how the brain worked to produce conscious-ness puts into perspective the responses to brain death after 1968, and the clinical challenges it faced. Later responses criticized brain death crite-ria as not engaging with the conceptual groundwork necessary to explain how brain, consciousness, and organism were related. These responses, characteristic of the bioethics literature on brain death, lose some cred-ibility around their claim to introduce a new conversation about the nec-essary conceptual groundwork when seen as yet another one of recurring attempts to do just that. The pre-1968 conversation was tied to testable methods in ways that the later bioethical conversation was often not. This underscores and helps explain the difficulties faced by the post-1968 criti-cal community to make instrumental use of their conceptual critique to learn more, to improve care, or to focus on the sort of core questions about what nature means and what science can do—questions that Jonas, and also Beecher, engaged.

As I suggested in Chapter Two, Jonas and Beecher—frequent exemplars of the oft-characterized divide between medical facts and ethical values that ostensibly called for bioethics—were similarly engaged with the proj-ect of how to take on the limits of dualism and to source values in nature. Beecher, though, saw no credible path of action coming from Jonas's and others' various critiques of the hubris reflected in setting man apart from nature via medical technologies. The neuroscientific study of conscious-ness briefly reviewed here, and especially the next chapter's analysis of its use in medical settings, are as yet underused opportunities to historically trace how medical facts might help broker and operationalize that project.

Jasper and Penfield, along with Cobb, were supported by the Rockefeller Foundation in a funding initiative intended to no less than do battle with that dualism—to unite psychiatry with medicine. The aim was for the neurosciences to describe brain function in ways that could be used to solve problems. For these clinicians and researchers, the actionability of some of the new models of how the brain worked was a key attraction. Restricting consciousness to a small part of the subcortical brain lent itself to a more targeted experimental approach. "This notion of the whole brain acting as a whole is, to my thinking and experimenting, rather sterile," remarked Jasper. "It gives us no possible conception of a real mechanism of integration. It leaves us completely without experimental approach to these problems."[53] EEG lent tangibility to brain action that could be translated into other experimental programs and then into potentially therapeutic action.

The complex link between these experimental paradigms and their actual use through the work of medicine can be seen in how the structures of the lower brain were described not only as parts of consciousness in terms, for example, such as in selecting among an array of sensations and ordering the sequence and objects of attention, but also as the building blocks of emotional experience, and in what those distinctions even meant. After reducing consciousness to snapshots of awareness, why not explain the dimensional and personal aspects of consciousness within these same events? Penfield, for example, elaborated on the emotional regulatory functions of temporal lobes, whose role in storing memories and mediating emotion was included in his centrencephalic ensemble. Philip Bard and Martin Macht also associated emotion more closely with these structures. They described the ability of decerebrate cats to roam freely, displaying stereotypically aggressive postures or other seemingly emotional reactions which, as Bard and Macht demonstrated, were only *pseudo*-affective—only having the outward form or appearance of an emotional experience. But at the 1959 CIBA Symposium, when Magoun asked them whether they therefore felt emotions could be localized to the brainstem or midbrain, Bard responded by raising a point central to later debates over brain death and to the comparisons of anencephalic, persistently vegetative, and brain-dead patients in those debates: "I am not prepared to say whether a decerebrate animal possesses subjective experience or not; *we have no way of telling that*" (emphasis mine).

Others seemed to be suggesting that the evidence indicated that they did have a way "of telling that." Penfield described how cortical stimulation can lead to vocalizations of crying while the patient reported not actually feeling sad, implying that the cortex provided just the form, and not the substance, of emotion. Magoun made this explicit: "If this were a response evoked by stimulating the cortex, I would not expect it to be associated with an affective experience." Chimed in Penfield: "I think the cortex is utilizing the mechanism in the brainstem."[54]

By the late 1950s, several summary reviews, conferences, and textbooks appeared that reflect the established presence of RAS as a key focus of research into brain function and consciousness, including Magoun's book *The Waking Brain*.[55] The "real significance" of EEG patterns "in terms of intra-cortical activity and of behavior" was "not completely known as yet." How much RAS was an active "director of attention with the actual work of consciousness" as opposed to a passive, though necessary, relay for attention, remained in dispute.[56] The process of establishing boundaries and differentiating roles between RAS in particular and associated midbrain structures, especially the thalamus and other midbrain centers, was often inconsistent. Thus, despite generating great creativity and opportunity, the value of EEG for clarifying the functional correlates of cortical activity was mixed.[57] While an appreciation of arousal and selective attention sequencing and coordination for consciousness was a lasting contribution of this work, it soon faded as a central aspect of consciousness studies, replaced by other methods of mapping the recruitment and activity of brain regions. But, during the 1950s and 1960s, the EEG and the map of consciousness it suggested provided critical working knowledge for several neurologists—Schwab and Adams prominently among them—to describe and manage patients in coma. The ambiguity of Bard's response, yet the repeatedly confirmed and tangible connections between brainstem and cortex, together lent confidence, but also the "whole brain" scope, to the eventual criteria, reinforced through experience with its use in care.

CLINICAL CHALLENGES TO THE LAB

How readily were ideas based on EEG recordings from brain-lesioned cats applied to cases like the following reported in 1952?

> A schoolgirl... [with] a sudden episode in which she lost consciousness for an hour, simultaneously she developed the further ocular signs and marked rigidity (recalling the decerebrate state... in subsequent months, had three essentially similar attacks... in each there was excessive sleepiness of several days' duration... Magoun and his school argue from [their] results that Bremer's conception is no longer tenable unless the concept of deafferentation be enlarged to include the reticular formation in its scope... by offering a constant background excitation directed towards the hemispheres... It is a speculation to be proved or disproved by pathological study.[58]

Such speculation caught the attention of leaders of twentieth-century neurology. Hugh Cairns addressed this topic in the Victor Horsely Memorial Lecture, which also appeared in the medical journal *Brain* in 1952.[59] He credited Moruzzi and Magoun's work for forcing a change in ideas regarding the residence of consciousness in the cortex, and for the rejection of Jackson's belief that it was centered there: "However... I must make clear what degree of 'consciousness' I consider is possible in the brain-stem and thalamus. The evidence, which is far from complete, comes from *human anencephalic and hydrocephalic monsters* who survive long enough to develop reactions."[60] Cairns noted that these patients, one surviving four decades, were able to eat, have preferences, go through sleep cycles, and show alertness, all with brainstems that functioned with only some or no remaining cortex. If coma did occur, it at times resembled sleep behaviorally and electroencephalographically, though without arousal; while at other times it appeared as something different, an unresponsiveness distinct from normal sleep. It was not clear then how a centrencephalic or reticular consciousness was appreciable or knowable in such patients and, consequently, whether Magoun's question to Bard and Macht was answerable or not. The relationship between RAS, cortex, and other regions and functions could be observed and mapped, but the translation of that mapping into conclusions about experience in general, or the anencephalic's experience in particular, was still elusive and may always be. Was Fessard's "experienced integration" enough of a phenomenon to be considered human consciousness?

Percival Bailey surveyed the implications of EEG-based research for treatment and patient care in his1955 presidential address before the American Neurological Association.[61] Bailey, a leading figure in early to mid-twentieth-century neurology,[62] remarked that Penfield's centrencephalon "may be more fundamental...more concerned with the primitive emotions, but the cerebral cortex (Jackson) is the highest level of the nervous system, the crowning glory of *Homo sapiens*." Consciousness boils down to the cortical "kaleidoscopic play which we call the mind." Consciousness without the cortex "must lead as dim and tenuous an existence as that of the shades in Hades. The cerebral cortex alone is capable of that bewildering play of intricate mental processes which is characteristic of human mentality."[63] Penfield's or Lindsley's "integration" was different from Bailey's. For the latter, brainstem (or thalamic) integration merely supported consciousness, whereas Penfield might consider this integration central to a concept of consciousness.

Citing a case of akinetic mutism of one year's duration with a completely absent EEG but diffusely injured neocortex, Bailey concluded, "It now appears that consciousness cannot be localized in the brainstem. It seems that one could no more localize consciousness than any other function of the nervous system. It must be looked upon as a machine."[64] In this case, holism and mechanism reinforced each other. Consciousness was present everywhere, and thus could be disrupted in a myriad of ways. The machine was not a pluripotential whole, like Lashley's, but at least a functionally unified one. Moruzzi and Magoun found "a regulating control" of reticular formation over cortex; Jasper revealed how the thalamus was included in that mechanism; and Bremer showed how the cortex also exerted influence over how these lower structures worked. This was how Bailey briefly summarized the state of EEG work on consciousness, attention, and awareness, at the time when Schwab first used EEG to support turning off a respirator. Bailey used that data to show just how dubious any localization of consciousness was. However, if consciousness was specifically understood as willful action and self-understanding, it remained in the cortex.

These distinctions began to matter at the bedside, and not just to Schwab. In another case report published in 1952, a five-year-old girl operated on for congenital hip displacement had a cardiac arrest mid-operation. She was given open cardiac massage and an intracardiac epinephrine injection with successful resuscitation after about five minutes. For decades, five minutes had been well known as a critical time window for cortical nerve cell survival. Almost two hours later, the EEG

"was practically a flat line, unmarked by any significant activity...At that time the patient was breathing spontaneously. Two hours and forty minutes after the accident, bursts of high amplitude and mixed frequency were noted in the EEG...The patient eventually died seventeen hours after the anoxic episode."

It does not appear that she was placed on a respirator. This girl was included as one case in a report of six cardiac arrests during operations. Two had flat EEGs and both died, leading to the tentative conclusion that "it seems to us that the EEG could be of some value in determining the prognosis after episodes of cerebral anoxia."[65]

Cardiac arrests in the operating room were an initial opportunity to connect EEG changes, prognoses, and mechanisms of injury and recovery.[66] Initially, however, conclusions as to the significance of EEG changes in coma, in particular a "flat-line," were cautious:

Recovery without evidence of residual abnormalities is possible from almost any type or degree of electroencephalographic disorder.

However, if the electroencephalographic activity has continued flat for over four hours there is a strong presumption that this cortical damage may not be completely reversible.[67]

Intensive care for life support was still new at this time. By 1950 the use of respirators was still limited, as was active cardiac massage and cardiac stimulatory medication for patients with cardiac arrest.[68] A small cadre of experts in coma emerged after expanded use of more mobile and effective positive pressure respirators for polio in particular, as described earlier, in the Danish epidemic of polio in the early 1950s. Many of the leaders of this successful public health effort founded some of the first "intensive care units." Beyond diseases of the respiratory mechanism, such as polio and myasthenia gravis, they spread the use of respirators to management of head trauma, cardiac arrest, respiratory illness, postoperative care, and so on.

In 1959, several papers by French investigators appeared that described a unique form of coma for which medical intervention was considered futile. Mollaret and Goulon coined the subsequently widely repeated term *coma dépassé*, or "beyond coma," to describe this state. In a continuous scale of comas—separated by degree of impaired responsiveness to the environment including reflexive, vegetative, and basic metabolic functions (respiration, circulation, thermal regulation)—*coma dépassé* was at an extreme end, absent all functions, the "total abolition of the vegetative functions of life."[69] This condition was found to have widespread necrosis—the essential effacement of the normal cellular components of the brain—as its pathology.[70] Jouvet argued that isoelectric EEGs could "permit the affirmation of the death of cortical and diencephalic formations" and suggest futility of further treatment.[71] Fischgold and Mathis published a review of 155 coma patients that attempted to find associations between clinical signs and EEG. Fischgold had been studying EEG and coma since at least the 1940s, and had devised the numbered (I through IV) scale of increasing severity of coma used by Jouvet. Stage IV described disruption of vegetative functions, the need for artificial life support, isoelectric EEG, and 100 percent mortality.[72]

That description, "*beyond* coma," is only comprehensible within the preceding decades of work on EEG and consciousness. *Coma dépassé* truly went beyond the nimble mechanisms or desynchronization paradigms with which Jouvet was so familiar. Those moving parts were gone. To these observers, *coma dépassé* described the end of discernible function of the nervous system as they understood it. It was beyond anything that had before appeared with beating heart and expanding lungs. Yet *coma dépassé* did not immediately translate into death. In part, this was because not all experts accepted the opinion of the authors that *coma dépassé* represented the absolute nonfunctioning of the brain, let alone the nervous system. Schwab's work was part of a process that unfolded over decades to capture and verify what the loss of these electrical signals meant.

Fred Plum—who emerged in the early 1960s as an international authority in coma—also became curious as to which signs reliably captured the degree of both nervous system and brain function loss in these patients. Plum authored the first comprehensive manual for the examination of the comatose patient, *The Diagnosis of Stupor and Coma*, which was published in 1966.[73] Working with polio patients at a respiratory care unit he had developed in Seattle, Washington, Plum became an expert in the management of hypoxia and respiratory insufficiency.[74] He then began admitting head trauma patients and others unable to breathe on their own into his convalescent polio unit, as the other hospital departments offered no similar intervention. The concentration of respirator use and expertise further expanded its application to a wide range of otherwise rapidly lethal conditions. But soon thereafter, by the mid-1950s, concern appeared in medical journals about sustaining otherwise unsalvageable patients in coma.

At the international meeting of transplant physicians and jurists sponsored by the CIBA foundation in 1966, several European transplant centers revealed that they were each using fairly comparable criteria with which to harvest organs from patients. They did so bolstered by the fact that at autopsy the brains and spinal cords of potential donors were similar to nervous systems in corpses over a week old.[75] This physical appearance was a striking and repeatedly invoked proof of brain death, the confirmation of a nonfunctioning brain. Beecher's friend and Committee member Joseph Murray commented at the CIBA gathering:

> I knew they were dead because I'd be waiting for them, I'd stop the post-mortem by taking out the kidneys, but I'd hang around for the rest of the post-mortem, and by the time they took the skull off the brain was just, uh, like oatmeal, no sulci, nothing there, just gone. So, I knew the patient had been really dead, in essence, long before we harvested the organ.[76]

But what were external, reliable signs of such extensive death of the brain that didn't require an autopsy to see? Many observers, including Fischgold, felt Mollaret and Goulon's coma dépassé might not mean irreversibility of brain damage, let alone death of the body, but was a particular state whose prognostic meaning could vary.[77]

So by 1968, at the threshold of defining brain death, one group of neurologists wrote that "the neurologist today appears practically without useful semiotic elements" to predict outcome in traumatic coma. Locating the level of the lesion through physical examination "does not reveal any prognostic meaning."[78] Part of this confusion lay in reconciling physical findings (i.e., unresponsiveness) and EEG findings; even patients with severe coma and extensive central nervous system loss at autopsy could still have EEG activation or reactivity.[79] Thus, while one review of almost two hundred cases of comatose patients with EEG found that "at times the isoelectric record...will raise the issue of the advisability for continued efforts to maintain life," EEG findings and physical findings still had to be interpreted in the context of each other: "When there is a marked discrepancy between the clinical and electrical signs—i.e., a relatively normal record with normal reactivity in a deeply comatose patient—the EEG should suggest a brain stem lesion."[80] But what did *that* suggest? Doubt and uncertainty about what EEG was describing captured a key problem for the EEG lab: Did the electric window into coma provide a picture of the status of mechanisms of consciousness and/or brain function, or was

it simply an indication of the extent of cell death from which those inferences about brain function could not yet reliably be made?

So, as Schwab started to gather material for what would be a series of
studies in the 1960s for his criteria, the "flat line" was still without stable meaning. In large part, this was because of inconsistent definition, as
some took flat line to simply mean low amplitude, which explained why
"10 percent of all adults" were described as having flat-line EEGs the year
the flurry of French reports appeared.[81] Fischgold reflected the feelings of
many when asserting that:

> "Flat EEG trace" does not signify death of the brain...but does have
> prognostic significance if it persists for hours or days in a subject who
> is at normal body temperature in the absence of anesthesia...Thus,
> prolonged electrical silence of the EEG, although it does not
> necessarily signify death of brain cells, acquires a grave prognosis.[82]

Through the 1950s and 1960s, some physicians increasingly raised questions about the connections between EEG and consciousness, and the significance of absent electrical activity. One patient could be reported to
have a "flat electroencephalogram" for twenty-eight days and eventually
fully recover.[83] Another, with atrophy of most of the reticular substance,
had a relatively normal EEG despite quadriplegia and absent response to
painful stimuli.[84] A published review of five coma patients concluded that
"our observations seem to justify the assumption that no one established
relationship exists between the intensity of coma and the recorded cere-
bral-electrical activity."[85] The authors tried to reconcile their findings with
the patterns of lesions in the cats of EEG brainstem researchers. Some
patients fit those patterns while others did not. Given the complexities of
the tiny universe of the pontine and midbrain space, perhaps "the nervous
structures involved in the regulation of the electroencephalographic activity and in the mechanism which gives rise to the state of consciousness
are different or that these structures have different functional activities."[86]

In another case, a patient with a brain stem infarct had a waking EEG but
was unresponsive to stimulation and demonstrated partial loss of cranial

nerve reflexes. This situation seemed to resemble cat experiments in which, at a particular midbrain transection, electrocortical activity and actual apparent awareness appeared to become disconnected, as they did here.[87] Similar findings in cats that showed persistent desynchronized unresponsiveness with transection at the midpontine pretrigeminal level generated interest and curiosity.[88] Desynchronization, usually associated with alertness, could apparently persist in cats without a synchronizing mechanism. Similar findings were detected in some unfortunate humans: "The question arises whether the patients and animals with such midpontine lesions are really conscious or not. Although ocular movements of the midpontine cats are suggestive of wakefulness this does not necessarily prove that the animals actually are conscious."[89] Magoun's question circled back to the bedside.

Patients with "akinetic mutism" especially seemed to resemble Bremer's cat transection experiments. The term itself is attributed to a description in a paper by Cairns of a patient in 1941:

> The patient sleeps more than normally, but he is easily aroused. In the fully developed state he makes no sound and lies inert, except that his eyes regard the observer steadily...Despite his steady gaze, which seems to give promise of speech, the patient is quite mute...Oft-repeated commands may be carried out in a feeble, slow and incomplete manner, but usually there are no movements of a voluntary character; no restless movements, struggling or evidence of negativism. Emotional movement is also in abeyance. A painful stimulus produces reflex withdrawal...[if] the stimulus is sustained, slow feeble voluntary movement may occur...but usually without tears, noise or other manifestations of pain or displeasure. The patient swallows readily, but has to be fed.[90]

Autopsy study of akinetic patients found extensive pontine and variable midbrain lesions, marring but not completely destroying the RAS:

> As a result of the partial destruction of the reticular formation, the reticular activating system may energize the neuronal activity derived

from external or internal stimuli to a degree sufficient to maintain movements of the eyes but not sufficient to maintain a degree of awareness permitting an intellectual command to be understood.[91]

The explanatory value and limits of "electricocentric life" developed substantially between Schwab's first observations with Brickley in 1941, to the Report in 1968. Severely comatose patients at MGH called for methods to "see" the seemingly inaccessible status of brain function in terms of the possibility for consciousness, the sustainability of physiological survival, and the permanence of either. EEG was a tangible window on the comatose brain, but also became central to efforts to develop those methods because of three results of these decades of EEG research. First was an empirical warehouse upon which to believe that EEG as a technology captured mechanisms that were reliably reproduced and had certain correlates to functioning of brain regions,; second, a working set of models and vocabulary to use to interpret but therefore to also test against more common clinical ways of knowing such as neurological and physical examinations; and third, to have models that also had problems—that highlighted key unanswered questions that shaped the scope of work and the limits and cautions in the use of these signs. Which mattered more—cortical EEG activity or brainstem function? Loss of working consciousness, of arousal mechanism, or overall loss of functioning brain cell mass? Was, as the Macy participant asked, "an isolated cortex useless to an animal"?

In his use of EEG to advise colleagues about continuing treatment and refine his criteria, Schwab had to consider—and his work was framed by—these questions. The prevailing position of the Committee was that the most reliable determination of certain incapacity for consciousness and brain function that could be drawn from this research and clinical experience lay in what would come to be referred to as the "whole brain" criteria. This whole brain position was not itself a conceptual or ethical position, yet it described the conditions that Beecher considered to risk unethical experiment and incoherent acts of commission. It was not adopted as a metaphorical stand-in for a commitment to a certain philosophy of mind or to the relative value of consciousness to personhood, yet it did use accumulated experimental and empirical findings that resulted from testing or elaborating such ideas. The criteria would later be criticized as being conceptually underdeveloped, and offering little or no empirical support. But the "whole" approach instead reflects a typical building of medical facts from these sources.

In the context of managing these new kinds of comatose patients, EEG research could identify for Schwab and his colleagues only the *scope* of brain mechanisms to confirm as having failed in order to render the demise of the capacity for consciousness, but could not as yet reliably specify with adequate consensus and patient care experience the more specific part(s) of that mechanism that did so. Schwab could also only credibly use criteria that included a coincident set of signs of the body's physiologic demise in these patients. The whole formulation allowed both, and had to allow for both. Within this point of view, deep within the building, testing, and use of medical knowledge in response to the severely comatose, such criteria described a set of tangible movements lost in death, as tangible as the loss of heartbeat.

NOTES

1. Robert S. Schwab, *Electroencephalography in Clinical Practice* (Philadelphia: WB Saunders Co., 1951): 158–59.
2. Robert S. Schwab, "Manuscript Outline for Book Proposal, 'Medico-Legal Aspects of Cerebral Death,'" 2. I am grateful for this and other papers belonging to Dr. Schwab obtained from his widow, Joan Schwab. This outline is undated, but likely circa 1970–72. Here Schwab also remarks that since 1954 "over 300 situations have arisen in our hospital where the presence or absence of an electroencephalogram is requested and if absent, and there is no breathing or reflexes, the patient can be declared dead. In these cases, 200 brains have been worked up in considerable detail and all of these cases showed marked dissolution and loss of structure," 3.
3. Schwab, "Manuscript Outline."
4. Robert S. Schwab, "The clinical application of electroencephalography," *Medical Clinics of North America* (September 1941): 1477–89.
5. Schwab, *Electroencephalography in Clinical Practice*.
6. Schwab, "Manuscript Outline," 2.
7. Robert Schwab, "The measurement of bodily currents," *Electrical Engineering* 60 (1941): 919–23, 922.

8. S. A. Kinnier Wilson, "On decerebrate rigidity in man and the occurrence of tonic fits," *Brain* 43 (1920): 220–68; 223–24; 226–27.

9. Sherrington, "Decerebrate rigidity and reflex co-ordination of movements," *Journal of Physiology* 22 (1897): 319.

10. Richard V. Lee, "Cardiopulmonary resuscitation in the eighteenth century: A historical perspective on present practice," *Journal of the History of Medicine* (October 1972): 418–33.

11. Astley Cooper, "Some experiments and observations on tying the carotid and vertebral arteries, and the pneumogastric, phrenic, and sympathetic nerves," *Guy's Hospital Report* 1 (1836): 457–75.

12. Librio Gomez and F. H. Pike, "The histological changes in nerve cells due to total temporary anemia of the central nervous system," *The Journal of Experimental Medicine* 11 (1909): 257–66, 257.

13. H. N. Simpson and A. J. Derbyshire, "Electrical activity of the motor cortex during cerebral anemia," *American Journal of Physiology* 109 (1934): 99.

14. H. K. Beecher, F. K. McDonough, and A. Forbes, "Effects of blood pressure changes on cortical potentials during anesthesia," *Journal of Neurophysiology* 1 (1938): 324–31; O. Sugar and R. W. Gerard, "Anoxia and brain potentials," *Journal of Neurophysiology* 1 (1938): 558–72.

15. E. D. Adrian and H. C. Matthews, "The Berger rhythm: potential changes from the occipital lobes in man," *Brain* 4, no. 57 (1934): 355–85.

16. For example, see a review by Morton A. Rubin, "The distribution of the alpha rhythm over the cerebral cortex of normal man," *Journal of Neurophysiology* 1 (1938): 313–23.

17. Otniel E. Dror, "Techniques of the brain and the paradox of emotions, 1880–1930," *Science in Context* 14, no. 40 (2001): 643–60.

18. David Milett, "Hans Berger: from psychic energy to the EEG," *Perspectives in Biology and Medicine* 4, no. 44 (Autumn 2001): 522–42.

19. Roger Smith, "Representations of mind: C. S. Sherrington and scientific opinion, c. 1930–1950," *Science in Context* 14, no. 4 (2001): 511–39.

20. G. Moruzzi and H. W. Magoun, "Brain stem reticular formation and activation of the EEG," *EEG and Clinical Neurophysiology* 1 (1949): 455–73.

21. The reticular activating system was generally considered a collection of highly interconnected nerve fibers extending from the first section of the brainstem distinguishable from the top of the spinal cord, the medulla, through the next section, a "bulb"-like appearing pons, and into the midbrain. However, as will be discussed, there was also a system of fibers extending from the region of important nuclei further rostral (towards the head), the thalamus, with the cortex, the cerebral hemispheres often referred to as the *thalamic reticular system*. Connections between these two systems were a source of great interest and productive of varying hypotheses of the nature of arousal and consciousness, and "reticulum" was often used to describe both systems or parts of them. These terms were further complicated by the finding of regions within these areas that seemed to have more particular functions, and the literature frequently included reasonable complaints that general comments about "the reticulum" nonspecifically referred to the general region

while perhaps describing more local effects. For characterizing the uses of these regions in reorienting versions of consciousness, the more general terms suffice.

22. D. B. Lindsley, L. W. Bowden, and H. W. Magoun, "Effect upon the EEG of acute injury to the brain stem activating system," *EEG and Clinical Neurophysiology* 1 (1949): 475–86, 483.

23. Morruzzi and Magoun, "Brainstem reticular formation and activation of the EEG," 468.

24. Among the work that factored in this discussion were Hess, *American Journal of Physiology* 90 (1929): 386; S. W. Ranson, "Somnolence caused by hypothalamic lesions in the monkey," *Archives of Neurology and Psychiatry* 41 (Chicago, 1939): 1–23; Robert S. Morison and Edward W. Dempsey, "A study of thalamico-cortical relations," *American Journal of Physiology* 135 (1942): 281–92; Dempsey and Morison, "The production of rhythmically recurrent cortical potentials after localized thalamic stimulation," *American Journal of Physiology* 135 (1942): 293–300; Dempsey and Morison, "The interaction of certain spontaneous and induced cortical potentials," *American Journal of Physiology* 135 (1942): 301; H. Jasper, J. Hunter, and R. Knighton, "Experimental studies of thalamocortical systems," *Transactions of the American Neurological Association* 73 (1948): 210–12; Herbert Jasper, "Diffuse projection systems: the integrative action of the thalamic reticular system," *EEG and Clinical Neurophysiology* 1 (1949): 405–20. Hess's work on the thalamus was explicitly tied by his son and co-workers to the agenda of moving cortical function to these subcortical areas in K. Akert, P. Koella and R. Hess, "Sleep produced by electrical stimulation of the thalamus," *American Journal of Physiology* 168 (1952): 260–67: "There have been numerous reports by Hess on the production of sleep in cats by electrical stimulation of the thalamus. These sprang from a concept developed in 1924 that the functional activity ('*Reactionsbereitschaft*') of the cerebral cortex is regulated by subcortical centers," 260. However, it is important to note that Hess and Ranson's prior work on the hypothalamic areas and supposed mechanisms of sleep were related to a view that part of the brain mediated the visceral stimuli shaping emotion, and thus when stimulated caused arousal. Thus, the elaborated roles of the thalamic areas in EEG research were ironically at first closely tied to afferentation models. They were also influenced by a prior fascination among earlier neurological investigators with animal, vegetative, and primitive influences on higher functioning, as suggested in the references to Reichardt's work below. All of this is to note the shifting interplay and iterative use of concept and experiment in the neuroscience of consciousness that the medical literature has actually long incorporated. As I will elaborate further, the focus of bioethical critique on the conceptual aspects of these sorts of facts further separated, rather than more usefully integrated this sort of iteration.

25. Herbert Jasper, "Diffuse projection systems: the integrative action of the thalamic reticular system," *EEG and Clinical Neurophysiology* 1 (1949): 405–20, 418.

26. Martin Reichhardt, "Hirnstamm und Psychiatrie," *Monatsschrift für Psychiatrie und Neurologie* 68 (1908): 470–506. (Translation in "Brain and Psyche," trans. F. I. Wertham, *Journal of Nervous and Mental Diseases* 70 (1929): 390–96.)

27. W. G. Walter, G. M. Griffith, and S. Nevin, *British Medical Journal* i (1939): 107.

28. Lindsley et al., "Effect upon the EEG," 485.

29. C. Judson Herrick, *The Thinking Machine*, 2nd ed. (Chicago: University of Chicago Press, 1932 [1929]).

30. Walter B. Cannon, "The James-Lange theory of emotions: a critical examination and alternative theory," *American Journal of Psychology* 39 (1927): 106–24, and idem "Again the James-Lange and the thalamic theories of emotion," *The Psychological Review* 38, no. 4 (July 1931): 281–95.

31. W. R. Hess, "Biological Order and Human Society," in *Biological Order and Brain Organization: Selected Works of W.R. Hess*, ed. K. Akert (Berlin: Springer-Verlag, 1981): 3–15. This originally appeared as "Kollektive Ordnung in biologischem Aspekt in: Festschrift Max Huber (Late President of the International Red Cross) – Vom Krieg und Frieden (Zurich: Schulthess, 1944): 151–72.

32. See, for example, Christopher Lawrence and George Weisz, eds., *Greater Than the Parts: Holism in Biomedicine 1920–1950* (New York: Oxford University Press, 1998); Anne Harrington, *Reenchanted Science: Holism in German Culture from Wilhelm II to Hitler* (Princeton: Princeton University Press, 1996).

33. Louise H. Marshall and Horace W. Magoun, eds., *Discoveries in the Human Brain: Neuroscience Pre-history, Brian Structure and Function* (Tatowa, N.J.: Humana, 1998).

34. Wilder Penfield, "The cerebral cortex in man: the cerebral cortex and consciousness," *Archives of Neurology and Psychiatry* 40, no. 3 (September 1938): 415–42, 441–42.

35. Transcripts of these meetings were collected as Harold A. Abramson, ed., *Problems of Consciousness*, transactions of a conference sponsored by the Josiah Macy Jr. Foundation (NY: Corlies, Macy and Co, Inc.): vol. 1 (1951) for March 20–21, 1950 meeting; vol. 2 (1951) for March 19–20, 1951 meeting; vol. 3 (1952) for March 10–11, 1952 meeting; vol. 4 (1954) for March 29–31 meeting; vol. 5 (1955) for March 22–24, 1954 meeting.

36. While not one of the more active participants, Beecher generally spoke of the need for measurable indices of function or behavior for study of consciousness, and of the need to avoid researching subjective qualities. That conclusion was likely reinforced by his claims about the efficacy of pain medications, as discussed in Chapter Two. Beecher also maintained a friendly correspondence with Moruzzi, and each hosted the other. Beecher Papers, Box 2, folder 37.

37. Alexander Barry in "Closing Remarks," in *Problems of Consciousness*, vol. 5, ed. Harold A. Abramson (1955): 155–61, 160.

38. Nathaniel Kleitman, in discussion of his presentation chapter "The Role of the Cerebral Cortex in the Development and Maintenance of Consciousness," in *Problems of Consciousness*, vol. 5, ed. Harold A. Abramson (1955): 111–32, 122.

39. Stanley Cobb, *Borderland of Psychiatry* (Cambridge, MA: Harvard University Press, 1943), 100. For a biographic review of Cobb's career, see Benjamin V. White, *Stanley Cobb: A Builder of the Modern Neurosciences* (Boston: Francis A. Countway Library of Medicine/University Press of Virginia, 1984).

40. Henry Alsop Riley in "Discussion on papers by Drs. Von Bonin, Magoun, and Jasper and associates," in *Archives of Neurology and Psychiatry*, 67, no. 2 (February 1952): 167–71, 167.

41. This experiment and its pointing towards a centrencephalic model are most fully described in Wilder Penfield, "Mechanisms of voluntary movement," *Brain* 77, no. 1 (March, 1954): 1–17.

42. E. D. Adrian, *The Physical Background of Perception* (London: Oxford University Press, 1947).

43. A. E. Fessard, "Mechanisms of Nervous Integration and Conscious Experience," in *Brain Mechanisms and Consciousness*, ed. J. F. Delafresnaye (Oxford: Blackwell, 1954), 200–36, 202. In his preface to these remarks in the published version of the transactions, Fessard includes a line from Heidegger's *Being and Time*, "Der Sinn des Daseins ist die Zeitlichkeit," translated as "the whole sense of Being is Time". References to phenomenological writings appeared not infrequently throughout this physiological and scientific literature regarding the nature of consciousness, though not in a systematic enough way to draw firm conclusions about possible connections between interpreting physiological data and these descriptions of experience. Perhaps more detailed biographies of individuals like Jasper, Moruzzi, Magoun, Lashley, Penfield, and Fessard might be useful in sorting through connections between culture and modeling consciousness, in particular connections to other areas of philosophy. That interaction has potential to inform as well the overall interest in this book on reconsidering how to leverage and improve the sourcing of values from the unique perspective of medical facts.

44. Stanley Cobb, "On the nature and locus of mind," *Archives of Neurology and Psychiatry* 67, no. 2 (February 1952): 172–77, 176–77.

45. N. Weiner, *Cybernetics: or Control and Communication in the Animal and the Machine* (New York: John Wiley and Sons Inc., 1948).

46. Quoted in Cobb, "On the nature and locus of the mind," 174. See Mary Brazier, "A neuronal basis of ideas," *Dialectica* 4 (1950): 73.

47. Norbert Weiner, *I Am a Mathematician: The Later Life of a Prodigy* (Garden City, NY: Doubleday & Company, Inc., 1956), 269.

48. Ibid., 291.

49. Lily E. Kay, "From logical neurons to poetic embodiment of mind: Warren S. McCullogh's project in neuroscience," *Science in Context* 14, no. 4 (2001): 591–614, 593. See also Michael Arbib, "Warren McCullough's search for the logic of the nervous system," *Perspectives in Biology and Medicine* 43, no. 2 (Winter 2000): 193–216. For a biography of his important and eccentric colleague Walter Pitts, see Neil R. Smalheiser, "Walter Pitts," *Perspectives in Biology and Medicine* 43, no. 2 (Winter 2000): 217–26.

50. In the second edition of *Cybernetics*, Weiner essentially appends sections to his original work dealing with EEG phenomenon in a chapter on "Brain Waves and Self-Organizing Systems." *Cybernetics: or Control and Communication in the Animal and the Machine* (Cambridge: MIT Press, 1969), 181–203.

51. See, for example, F. H. George, *The Brain as a Computer* (New York: Pergamon Press, 1961).

52. K. S. Lashley, *Brain Mechanism and Intelligence: A Quantitative Study of Injuries to the Brain* (Chicago: University of Chicago Press, 1929), 173.

53. In "General Discussion," in *Brain Mechanisms and Consciousness*, J. F. Delafresnaye ed., 500.

54. Discussion in Philip Bard and Martin B. Macht, "The Behaviour of Chronically Decerebrate Cats," in *CIBA Foundation Symposium on the Neurological Basis of Behavior*, eds. G. E. W. Wolstenholme and Cecilia M. O'Connor (Boston: Little, Brown and Co., 1958): 55-75, 72-73.

55. H. W. Magoun, *The Waking Brain*, 2nd ed. (Springfield, Ill: Charles C. Thomas, 1963 [1958]); Herbert H. Jasper, et al., eds., *Reticular Formation of the Brain* (Boston: Little, Brown & Company, 1958); GianFranco Rossi and Alberto Zanchetti, "The brain stem reticular formation," *Archives Italiennes de Biologie* 9 (1957): 199-433.

56. Rossi and Zanchetti, "The brain stem reticular formation," 404, 463, and 404.

57. Giusseppe Moruzzi, review of "Reticular formation of the brain," *EEG and Clinical Neurophysiology* 11 (1959): 624-29.

58. Michael Jefferson, "Altered consciousness associated with brain-stem lesions," *Brain* 75 (1952): 55-67, 59, 66.

59. Hugh Cairns, "Disturbances of consciousness with lesions of the brain-stem and diencephalon," *Brain* 75, no. 2 (June 1952): 109-46.

60. Hugh Cairns, "Disturbances of consciousness with lesions of the brain-stem and diencephalon," 113.

61. Percival Bailey, "Concerning the localization of consciousness," *Transactions of the American Neurological Association* 80 (1955): 1-12.

62. Bonnie Ellen Blustein, "Percival Bailey and neurology at the University of Chicago, 1928-1939," *Bulletin of the History of Medicine* 66 (1992): 90-113.

63. Bailey, "Concerning the localization of consciousness," 9.

64. Ibid., 6.

65. Y. K. J. Gronqvist, Thomas Sheldon, and Albert Faulconer, "Cerebral anoxia during anesthesia: prognostic significance of electroencephalographic changes," *Annales chirurgiae et gynaecologiae Fenniae* 41 (1952): 149-59, 155-56, 158.

66. J. Weldon Bellville, Joseph Artusio, and Frank Glenn, "The electroencephalogram in cardiac arrest," *JAMA* 157, no. 6 (February 5, 1955): 508-10; J. Weldon Bellville and William S. Howland, "Prognosis after severe hypoxia in man," *Anesthesiology* 18, no. 3 (May-June 1957): 389-97.

67. Bellville and Howland, ibid., 396.

68. One early report of such aggressive intervention is in J. C. Fox Jr., "Restoration of cerebral function after prolonged cardiac arrest," *Journal of Neurosurgery* 6 (1947): 361, 1949. This paper is still cited in 1951 as the sole example of such resuscitative attempts for severe cerebral anoxia in a paper otherwise typical of period treatments of the subject in describing general typologies of different kinds of anoxic injury (e.g., "anoxic type," "anemic type," "stagnant type"), reiterating various theories about how this toxicity happens with a limited research base, and rehearsing well known relationships between limited time of complete anoxia and nerve cell death. See A. Theodore Steegmann, "Clinical aspects of cerebral anoxia in man," *Neurology* 1 (1951): 261-74.

69. P. Mollaret and M. Goulon, "Le Coma Dépassé," *Revue Neurologique* 101, no. 1 (1958): 3-15, 4.

70. P. Mollaret, Ivan Bertrand, and H. Mollaret, "Coma dépassé et nécroses nerveuses centrales massives," *Revue Neurologique* 101, no. 2: 116-39. A pathology research

literature would soon begin to develop, interested in the cellular events involved in the syndrome of a coma with loss of vegetative regulatory control. See W. Kramer, "From reanimation to deanimation," *Acta Neurologica Scandinavica* 39, no. 2 (1962): 139–53.

71. M. Jouvet, "Diagnostic Electro-sous-corticographique de la mort du systeme nerveux central au cours de certains comas," *Electroencephalography and Clinical Neurophysiology* 11 (1959): 805–8, 808.

72. H. Fischgold and P. Mathis, "Obnubilations, comas et stupeurs: 'Etudes Electroencephalographique." *EEG and Clinical Electroencephalography Suppl* 11 (1959), reported and abstracted in Daniel Silverman, "Retrospective study of EEG in coma," *Electroencephalography and Clinical Neurophysiology* 15 (1963): 486–503.

73. Fred Plum and Jerome B. Posner, *The Diagnosis of Stupor and Coma* (Philadelphia: FA Davis Co., 1966).

74. See, for example, Fred Plum and August Swanson, "Abnormalities in central regulation of respiration in acute and convalescent poliomyelitis," *AMA Archives of Neurology and Psychiatry* 80 (September 1958): 267–85.

75. See J. Hamburger in "Discussion" of the paper, "Organ transplants: practical possibilities," in *CIBA Foundation Symposium Ethics in Medical Progress—With Special Reference to Transplantation,* eds. G. E. W. Wolstenholme and Maeve O'Connor (Boston: Little, Brown, and Co., 1966): 65–77, 74. Hamburger was chief of the renal unit at Hopital Necker, Paris, and used criteria outlined by G. P. J. Alexandre, the head of renal transplantation at Hopital St. Pierre, Belgium, part of the University of Louvain. In addition to fixed dilated pupils, unresponsiveness, total areflexia, apnea, and a flat EEG, Alexandre added falling blood pressure, which required increased vasopressor drugs. With the latter, internal homeostasis was disappearing and thus patients meeting his criteria usually died on the respirator within hours. See *CIBA Foundation.,* 69–70. Reports from yet another French hospital in Lyon added to these criteria absence of cortical circulation. Murray was an active participant in these discussions and very familiar with these practices.

76. Joseph Murray, interview with the author, February 18, 1998.

77. See H. Fischgold in "Introduction-Utilization of EEG Signs of Cerebral Hypoxia During Open Heart Surgery," in *Cerebral Anoxia and the Electroencephalogram,* eds. Henri Gastaut and John Stirling Meyer (Springfield IL: Charles C Thomas, 1961), 229–30.

78. B. Bergamasco, L. Bergamini, and T. Doriguzzi, "Clinical value of the sleep electroencephalographic patterns in post-traumatic coma," *Acta Neurologica Scandinavica* 44 (1968): 495–511, 495.

79. A. Bricolo, A. Gentilomo, G. Rosadini, and G. F. Rossi, "Long-lasting post-traumatic unconsciousness," *Acta Neurologica Scandinavica* 44 (1968): 512–32; Alberto Fois, Erna L. Gibbs, and Frederic Gibbs, "'Flat' electroencephalograms in physiological decortication and hemispherectomy (recordings awake and asleep)," *EEG and Clinical Neurophysiology* 7 (1955): 130–34.

80. Daniel Silverman, "Retrospective study of EEG in coma."

81. A. Adams, "Studies on the flat electroencephalogram in man," *EEG and Clinical Electroencephalography* 11 (1959): 35–41, 40.

82. H. Fischgold, in discussion of Nenad Bokonjic, Fritz Buchtal, "Postanoxic uncon-sciousness as related to clinical and EEG recovery in stagnant anoxia and carbon monoxide poisoning," in *Cerebral Anoxia and the Electroencephalogram*, eds. Henri Gastaut and John Stirling Meyer, 118–27, 128.

83. E. Bental and U. Leibowitz, "Flat electroencephalograms during 28 days in a case of 'encephalitis,'" *EEG and Clinical Neurophysiology* 13 (1961): 457–60.

84. Arne Lundervold, Tormond Hauge, and Aagot Loken, "Unusual EEG in uncon-scious patient with brain stem atrophy," *EEG and Clinical Neurophysiology* 8 (1956): 665–70. See also Arne Lundervold, "Electroencephalographic changes in a case of acute cerebral anoxia unconscious for about three years," *EEG and Clinical Neurophysiology* 6 (1954): 311–15. Here, a thirteen-year-old boy with asphyxia went for two months without electrical activity on EEG, developed EEG responses to some stimuli at fifteen months, and showed seizure patterns over two years after. In this case, the author is puzzled as to what to call consciousness and how to describe it neurophysiologically. He offers Jackson, Jasper, and Magoun as possible helpful sources pointing to the frontal lobes, thalamus, and RAS, respectively, but leaves the question open and unresolved.

85. Carlo Loeb, Guido Rosadini, and G. F. Poggio, "Electroencephalograms dur-ing coma," *Neurology* 9 (1959): 610–18, 615. See also, with similar conclusions, Carlo Loeb, "Electroencephalographic changes during the state of coma," *EEG and Clinical Neurophysiology*, 10, no. 4 (November 1958): 589–606.

86. Loeb, Rosadini, and Poggio, "Electroencephalogram during coma," 618.

87. Gian Emilio Chatrian, Lowell E. White Jr., and Cheng-Mei Shaw, "EEG pattern resembling wakefulness in unresponsive decerebrate state following traumatic brain infarct," *EEG and Clinical Neurophysiology* 16 (1964): 285–89.

88. C. Batini, G. Moruzzi, M. Palestini, G.F. Rossi, and A. Zanchetti, "Persistent patterns of wakefulness in the pretrigeminal midpontine preparation," *Science* 128 (1958): 30–32. These experiments are described in some detail by Antonio Damasio in *The Feeling of What Happens* (1999). While updating understanding of these findings in light of hypotheses regarding the functions of the particular nuclei cut, Damasio concludes also that despite wakefulness and possible atten-tion, even with "intact all of the structures necessary to implement the proto-self," one of Damasio's core aspects of consciousness served up by more subcortical structures, "whether or not normal consciousness would still be possible is a ques-tion that cannot be decided...and certainly will never be answered in humans." Antonio Damasio, *The Feeling of What Happens: Body and Emotion in the Making of Consicousness* (New York: Harcourt, Brace and Co., 1999), 257.

89. B. R. Kaada, W. Harkmark, and O. Stokke, "Deep coma associated with desynchro-nization in EEG," *EEG and Clinical Neurophysiology* 13 (1961): 785–89, 788

90. H. Cairns, et al., "Akinetic mutism with an epidermoid cyst of the third ventricle," *Brain* 64 (1941): 273–90, 273.

91. Humberto Craviato, Jacobo Silberman, and Irwin Feigin, "A clinical and patho-logic study of akinetic mutism," *Neurology* 10 (1960): 10–21, 20.

5

The Criteria II: The Working Brain and the Comatose Patient

"[Magoun's] The Waking Brain...with its appearance the brain of man and animals ceased to be regarded as a purely passive responding apparatus [but]...it did not attempt to analyse the fundamental forms of human concrete psychological activity."

—A. R. LURIA, *The Working Brain, 1973*

"I like my head. How about you? It lets me know I'm alive."

—BARNEY

Robert Schwab first advised colleagues to turn off a respirator in 1954, based upon EEG and clinical exam findings. The criteria he proposed for the Harvard Report, however, evolved through a series of studies, published through the 1960s, that looked at the outcomes of comatose patients. These studies, and the uses of EEG and examination to guide care for those with severe coma, drew in part upon EEG research on the "waking brain." Many commentators critical of the Harvard criteria faulted its lack of an empirical basis and failure to explicitly describe a concept of death. However, any assessment of the Report should include attention to the actual care of these patients at MGH, and to Schwab' s efforts to develop and use the criteria he presented to the Committee.

Schwab was clearly conversant with research and controversies surrounding the use of EEG to explain brainstem and subcortical mechanisms in brain function. He played a central role in the institutional growth and research base of electroencephalography. In 1937, at MGH, he established one of the first, if not the first EEG laboratory ever to be sited in a hospital.[1] He was a founding officer (secretary) of The American Society of Electroencephalography, which was established in 1947 with Jasper as its first president, a post Schwab would later assume. Schwab was also the founding managing editor of the journal *EEG and Clinical Neurophysiology*, through which much of the key work on establishing reticular and subcortical roles in central nervous function appeared.

Schwab did not use EEG in order to advise colleagues to end treatment simply because some mechanism of consciousness was no longer functioning. He wanted to solve a concrete problem for his colleagues: Could interobserver replicable findings indicate when these patients were no longer subjects for medical attention? The interaction of EEG and neurological research, expectations about extraordinariness of care, the specific capabilities and limitations of medical practice in the 1960s, and the behavior of the brain and the body under these circumstances contributed to the possibility that brain death was death. So was brain death a straightforward "mere" fact, or a contexted practice? Brain death, as a President's Council on Bioethics senior consultant put it, "is far from a mere social construct. It is a biologically well-grounded response to the lived phenomenon of the 'brain dead' patient."[2] Medical practices and the empirical strategies from which they emerge as "biologically well-grounded responses," have to be central to any serious look at social uses, benefits, and implications of these facts. But at the same time, and as I will argue in the following chapter, the social contingency and purposes of medical facts are also crucial to understanding them and bothering to use them. Later bioethics debates often simplified this complexity and took brain death out of its sources.

THE REPORT

Very little of the initial April 11 Report draft detailed the criteria of "irreversible coma" but where it did, it featured what Schwab referred to as his "triad" of symptoms describing brain death.[3] Two sections took on this task: "Definition of Irreversible Coma" by Beecher, and a subsequent section entitled "Characteristics of Irreversible Coma," which included material Beecher attributed to Schwab's work. These few paragraphs contain varying descriptions of the symptoms and signals the criteria were meant to cover. "Characteristics" described Schwab as a pioneer in using EEG to diagnose "brain death." In a subsequent "discussion," Beecher lamented using extraordinary means to sustain persons who had "no hope of recovery of consciousness" and stated that the definition of irreversible coma permitted removing extraordinary means with "death *to follow.*" He then observed that the "moment of death" is seen to "*coincide* with irreversible coma while the heart continues to beat." The April 11 draft was addressed to the "Committee to Define Irreversible Coma,"[4] while later notes and memoranda describe it as the as "Ad Hoc Committee to Examine the Definition of Brain Death" or "Ad Hoc Committee on Brain Death."[5] When presenting his autopsy study of ninety cases meeting his triad (a study which was cited in this early draft) at a scientific meeting during the Committee's tenure, Schwab remarked, "we say the time of death is the time the heart stops beating"[6] [emphases mine]. Although, as will be seen in MGH medical records, Schwab actually distinguished what he meant by "death" in several ways.

From the outset, then, the Report contained various ways to understand its opening claim that "our primary purpose is to define irreversible coma as a new criterion for death." The Report, especially in its earlier drafts, alternated between descriptions of a coma that predicted heart-based death and a coma that was death itself. While this became a focus of criticism in the decades following the appearance of the Report, this potential ambiguity, and its evolution in Report drafts, reflects an important moment in medical practice that needs to be understood—as does the discomfort it generated.

Brain death was, and is, bound up with both ontological and prognostic purposes: it describes death *and* its imminence. The conditions of death before dying brought the tasks of defining death and defining futility closer together, such that they were indistinguishable within the context of care as understood by those who first framed it, and within a set of attitudes described earlier around experimentation and medical knowledge. Commentators later sought to resolve this overlap of descriptive and prognostic purposes by crafting more careful conceptual distinctions between death and dying. As the Report most unambiguously stated, though, its starting point was technically narrower—to describe the "characteristics of a *permanently* non-functioning brain." That such a state meant death to these authors was by virtue of Beecher's pragmatism, Schwab's empiricism, and experience with comatose bodies in the hospital, which is the focus of this chapter.

Schwab responded to the April 11 draft by emphasizing that what the Committee was trying to do was to identify a particular form of irreversible coma that predicted death with certainty in the absence of life support. On his copy of the early Report draft that he sent to Beecher, he scribbled in his characteristically large hand that "it is not necessary to change definition of death to define Brain Death. If we establish the concept of irreversible coma with cessation of function at all levels of the CNS it will not be difficult…to withhold or discontinue [treatment.]"[7] Schwab initially argued that the Committee's focus on redefining death was not the right posture, strategically. The key function of the Report, he reasoned, was to define irreversible coma as a distinct and unique neurological entity, and assumed that the consequences of that definition would follow. Schwab shared (apparently at the prior Committee meeting) a confidential memorandum summarizing initial findings from what would be a widely quoted study conducted by the American EEG Society on EEG, survival, and coma that appeared the following year. He wrote to Beecher in May 1968 about the first set of what would be a review of over two thousand reports of EEG and coma outcomes. While over seven hundred reports had been gathered by that point, no patients with a "flat" EEG had survived. However, there were many "flat EEGs" that did not meet his full triad.[8] This seemed to underscore his own experience with varying presentations of isoelectric coma and to the potential confusion over what signs constituted irreversible and compete loss of brain function—an issue Schwab explored with colleagues for at least decade, as will be reviewed here.

The first order of business, then, was to get consistency and rigor around the description of this coma. In the memorandum to Beecher Schwab therefore advised, "Do not attempt to redefine death. Concentrate on agreement as to what constitutes *irreversible coma.*"[9] The medical records of the patients Schwab saw, and for whom he advised withdrawal of treatment, included many patients for whom care was discontinued based on reasons other than meeting this kind of criteria. So, discontinuation of care did not need this definition. But this kind of coma needed care to end. This coma was different and needed to be reliably distinguished in the ways it was different. His experience with patients, and the potential for confusion without informed and shared criteria as evidenced by this growing data set, led him to advise Beecher in his memorandum to stay focused on communicating a standard or guideline for definition of irreversible coma itself. His advice to Beecher did not mean he did not think it reflected death, but underscored how death was described in those details and so emphasized getting those details understood and accepted. Those details essentially boiled down to finding the full triad, a twenty-four hour duration of those findings, and the absence of confounding conditions (e.g., barbiturate overdose). It "may be too conservative but it will serve as a guideline."

Schwab offered detailed language in the next draft that built on the more sketchy April 11 version of the criteria under the "characteristics" section, which was essentially what Beecher copied as his gloss on Schwab's work from Eliasburg. The new proposed section, entitled "Details to Establish Irreversible Coma with no CNS Activity," brought together descriptions of apnea and nonresponsiveness (from an earlier section of the draft), and of flat EEG (from a later section) in order to more compactly describe Schwab's "triad" of "no movements or breathing," "no reflexes," and a "flat encephalogram." Beecher edited this section for style but not content; in the next draft that appears in the archives, this remained the only section detailing the actual criteria, until further edits were made by Adams in June.

In the interim, other changes by Beecher show that some of Schwab's overall comments rubbed off in edits that remained in the published version. The introductory sentence from the April "background" section stayed in, but was now preceded by a new sentence, a la Schwab, that read: "Irreversible coma can have many causes, but *we are concerned only with those comatose individuals who have no discernible central nervous system activity*."[10] This was the only italicized sentence in the published Report, as it was underlined by Beecher in his surviving manuscript. Schwab's triad itself then followed under the unchanged heading of "Characteristics of Irreversible Coma," and a new section called "Other Procedures" described how to inform family, nurses, and involved colleagues when the criteria were met. Only at this point, with some of the ambiguity of the prior drafts removed, did the subsequent drafts and final version of the Report state that "death is to be declared and then the respirator turned off."

Curran's "Death and the Law" section came next, followed by a new "discussion" section, and closed finally by a summary that contained the most explicit description in the Report of the underlying understanding of the mechanisms of consciousness. The "Summary" focused on detailing how "Cerebral, cortical and thalamic involvement are indicated by a complete absence of receptivity of all forms of sensory stimulation and a lack of response to stimuli and to inner need." This unresponsive and unreceptive state always has "coincident paralysis of brain stem and basal ganglionic mechanisms" with absent cranial and postural reflexes:

Involvement of the spinal cord, which is less constant, is reflected usually in loss of tendon reflexes…Of the brain stem–spinal mechanisms which are conserved for a time the vasomotor reflexes are the most persistent…[and are] responsible for the paradoxical state of retained cardiovascular function…in the face of widespread disorder of the cerebrum, brain stem and spinal cord.

All of these changes persisted into publication except for consequential additions by Adams, who edited Schwab's triad to better emphasize exceptions in case of the presence of depressant substances or medications, and to make more prominent and detailed (and perhaps redundant) the notion of unresponsivity. These edits reshuffled the substance of the first two legs of the triad into three. The first criteria was "Unreceptivity and Unresponsivity," which overlapped in terms of features of physical examination with the following two but provided a clarifying statement about the irreversible functional losses of the body at stake here—a formulation (unreceptivity, unresponsivity) not too far from that which, many decades later, continued to animate commentary over the underlying theory of death implicit in brain death. The criteria that followed were then "No Movement or Breathing," which described the need for apnea, properly tested, and no movements or responsiveness to stimuli. After that came "No Reflexes," which Adams also edited in detail to describe specific cranial and other reflexes. "Flat Encephalogram" thus became a fourth criteria, "of great confirmatory value."

Of note, Joseph Murray's suggested edits for the April 11 draft consisted primarily of pointing out references to "irreversible coma" and recommending either rewriting them so that only the word "death" be used, or else clearly indicating that the two terms were synonymous. This included a suggestion to change the first sentence to read simply that the report's purpose was to "define death." None of these suggestions were taken. However, between the June 3 and 7 drafts, Beecher did change the first sentence, from "our primary purpose here is to define irreversible coma," to "our primary purpose is to define irreversible coma as a new criteria for *pronouncing* death" [emphasis mine].

This formulation—that this coma pronounces but is not itself explicitly death—smoothed over much of the ambiguity, if not outright contradiction, in the original working drafts, but still presented to the world an interesting medical fact. Irreversible coma was indeed unique. It was a coma with "no discernible...activity," an as-if-dead state, allowing practices usually linked to a body absent of motion to now be associated with a body unable to experience and respond: a neurologically empty body. The writing of the Report resisted calling irreversible coma simply death, but at the same time made it an event which justified "pronouncing" death. And yet, while its title describes irreversible coma, the Report describes the Committee as determining "brain death."

The Report did not provide a worked out, consistent notion of death—or even of life. Why not Murray's edits? Why not black and white clarity, calling irreversible coma death? Why did Beecher instead add language about "pronouncing" death, implying (but not outright stating) the equation of irreversible coma with death itself? Press reports and subsequent discussions characterized the Report as defining death, and Beecher himself later regularly referred to it as such.

In these edits we witness a change wherein the boundaries of death, themselves coherent in the context of the limits of the medically possible, reflected how what was medically possible was itself increasingly shaped and experienced at the bedside with these patients by the limits of the nervous system. Conditions of death before dying required facing the implications of caring for individuals essentially absent a nervous system. The resulting ascendancy of nervous system function as a factor in "the calculus of suffering" wasn't *advocated*, it was described and *managed*.

In 1953, Raymond Adams was asked to examine and advise in the treatment of a housewife with a brain tumor. The neurological exam found "pupils fixed, equal at 3 mm...areflexic throughout including corneals. Extremities flaccid. No response to pinprick." She died early that night when she stopped breathing. A few years later, the same examination findings had different significances within the context of other findings that had become possible because of the respirator. What those findings meant and caused to happen, or caused people to think about, would change. Fixed pupils and areflexia were not simply "discovered" as "real" death. The fixed pupil and the nonresponsive reflex arc were physical events whose nature and significance were themselves changed by the respirator and by additional new methods for sustaining blood pressure and other vital functions.

Attention to these comatose patients paralleled their increasing presence in hospital care. Consider that in 1958 at MGH, sixty-six patients required ventilator support for more than twenty-four hours. By 1964, that number was 398.[11] Beecher realized the need to put individuals requiring "oxygen treatment" into a concentrated area in the late 1950s, as he recognized that the increasing expertise and labor required for the management of such patients was inefficiently dispersed through the hospital. Growing awareness of such inefficiency, and in particular the death of an MGH service chief's relative from myasthenia gravis (a paralyzing neurologic disorder), combined to secure resources for a dedicated respiratory unit. It opened at MGH in October of 1961 to specialize in the care of respirator-dependent patients.[12] This effort paralleled similar recognition by many hospitals of the challenges raised by growing numbers of these patients, accelerating concern by some within medicine about the aggressiveness that increasingly characterized this care. Those cared for in the MGH unit during the early to mid-1960s—when Schwab was particularly active pruning his criteria—did not, for the most part, fit the description of the "irreversibly comatose." It is hard to estimate how many patients did. Schwab reported that he tallied three hundred cases in which he was involved from 1954 to 1970, mostly during the 1960s.[13]

Schwab was not alone in wanting to draw lines and limits around the new technologies of intensive care at MGH. Neurosurgeon Hannibal Hamlin made the following argument:

Respirators and heart stimulators can maintain the look of life in the face of death while agonizing and expensive prolongation of false hope continues for all concerned. When the brain is so compromised, the EEG can signal the point of no return ... interpretation of the EEG should gain medical approval for legal pronouncement of human death.[14]

Hamlin reported that Schwab's criteria, as set forth in a 1962 paper, were used to end life support fifteen times at MGH. Presented at the American Electroencephalographic Society, that paper outlined the following criteria: absence of spontaneous respirations for one hour; no tendon reflexes or pupil reflexes; dilated pupils; no arousal to stimuli on EEG; an isoelectric

EEG for one hour; and no heart range change to eyeball pressure. Hamlin reported that ten patients had been diagnosed this way, seven "in the past two years."[15] The following year, additional experience with thirty-four more cases was presented.[16] In 1964, Hamlin announced to the national medical audience that Schwab, using these basic criteria, had "accepted responsibility with support of his colleagues for death pronouncement by EEG some 15 times during the past $2^{1/2}$ years. The experience," Hamlin went on, had "proved eminently satisfactory to all concerned, diminishing grief and anxiety for the family of the victim in a state of limbo, also relieving the travail and expense of skilled personnel, special equipment, and service."[17] William Sweet recalled that Hamlin may have made the connection for Schwab between his work on EEG correlates to nonsurvival and a legal process of defining death;[18] at least one newspaper account described Hamlin as having "set up a set of criteria for certifying brain death" with Schwab.[19] In his 1962 presentation, Schwab observed:

> The new cardiac stimulation, other techniques, and compact respirators, have made it increasingly possible to revive the apparently dead. Fortunate cases recover both respiratory and higher central nervous function as well as normal cardiac activity. This communication is not involved with these patients...In these cases a human heart-lung preparation results that may be viable for many days...In such cases the prolongation of cardiac circulation serves no purpose, is a tremendous financial and emotional stress to the relatives, and a severe demand on hospital personnel and equipment.[20]

Schwab also struck up a friendship with Sidney Rosoff, who was at that time an attorney for the Euthanasia Society of America and who would later become its president, as well as the president of the Hemlock Society, which advocated assisted suicide. When Schwab needed funds to support travel to (and participate in) the USSR Academy of Medical Sciences Symposium on Reanimation, held in Moscow from November 25–29, 1968, Rosoff facilitated access to funds from the Euthanasia Society.[21]

Schwab, said Rosoff, "was ahead of his time" and saw brain death as part of broader questions that needed more attention regarding patient preference about life support termination.[22] Rossof was co-author with Schwab of a 1967 paper, the one Curran commented on to Beecher, read before a later American Electroencephalographic Society gathering that reported on the use of the criteria at MGH for over 150 cases.[23] Schwab's interest in refining the criteria was to validate the ability to identify those beyond coma, not to advance transplant. Fred Plum, by then a world leader in the study of coma, recalled that his and his colleague's understanding of the Harvard Report, at the time of publication, was that it reflected an interest not in transplant but in the work he and others had grappled with for decades, on the implications of and mechanisms behind severe coma.[24] My own review of care at MGH, described further in the following pages, draws on medical records of 421 patients in coma who had EEGs performed by Schwab's EEG service during the decade before the Report's criteria for brain death were published (1958–1967). Seventy-one of these patients met what would later be established as the Harvard criteria for brain death. Interest in transplantation is not evident from these records. The issue of organ donation was documented for consideration for transplantation in the medical records of only two. In neither case were organs harvested. But the emerging utility, content, and purpose of the criteria, as well as the applicability and use of EEG and neurologic examination in the circumstances of this new irreversible coma, can be seen in these records.

THE PATIENTS

Growing and concentrated numbers of respirator-bound patients spurred several efforts to describe the examination, diagnosis, and prognosis of coma—most notably by Plum, as well as by C. Miller Fisher, then the director of MGH's Stroke Service.[25] Their work set the standard for neurological examination of comatose patients through the latter twentieth century.

Increased interest in the use of neurologic signs for clinical prognosis meant rethinking which neurologic signs mattered. Admitted in 1966 for a skull fracture, a twenty-nine-year-old mother of three is described as being revived from a cardiac arrest only to be "areflexic—anticipate EEG today will be without cortical activity and thus resuscitative measures should be abandoned." Schwab subsequently reported that her "tracing is flat," as were two repeat EEGs twenty-four hours and three days later, at which point such measures were abandoned. However, another patient in 1959 was similarly apneic, with absolutely no activity in any of her cranial nerves, no spinal reflexes, and no movement or responsiveness to any stimuli presented. In this case, resuscitation was vigorously attempted. One difference between these two patients was that the second woman overdosed on barbiturates, which might have only temporarily affected brain functions. Consensus over the importance of distinctions like these and their impact on the reliability and use of different neurological signs took work and cumulative experience, and even then were varyingly adopted in practice. Schwab—who was called upon by colleagues to assess coma with EEG, and was well versed in EEG-based research on brain function and consciousness—explored these questions. Which findings were reliably irreversible? What neurologic signs indicated that the brain no longer functioned? That treatment was no longer relevant to outcome?

MASSACHUSETTS GENERAL HOSPITAL RECORDS

The circumstances in which Schwab and his colleagues wrestled with these questions, and the patient histories that informed their studies, can be found in surviving medical records at MGH. Records for this review were identified through index card summaries of EEGs (performed by Schwab's MGH EEG service), which were available in the Department of Neurology archives and dated back to near the outset of Schwab's tenure at MGH. Preserved on microfilm, these brief summaries contained the results of approximately10,000 EEGs performed from 1958 through 1967, the decade preceding the Committee's work as well as the period during which Schwab used some of these cases to evaluate and revise his criteria. Of these summaries, most of which were routine studies done on outpatients, I selected all EEG reports that mentioned the word "coma." This yielded over six hundred medical record identifier numbers and of these, 421 medical records could be retrieved and reviewed.

These hospital records described patients with markedly poor prognoses but widely varying approaches to the determination of when care ended. Why were these EEG consults requested and how were they used? To start, in only 163 (39 percent) of these cases was the EEG even noted to have been read or reviewed by the patient's physician. The patterns of how EEGs were used, however, are consistent with discriminating and focused purposes that suggest that Schwab's irreversible coma, as his edits to Beecher also suggested, was perceived as a unique entity—one which presented challenges distinct from (though overlapping with) other decisions to remove care among those severely ill. I return to this detail as it becomes relevant to post-Report commentary, as it did to Beecher's early critics in Chapter 2. To those contemporaries of Beecher, the Committee was often described to simply be looking for a reasonable point to justify withdrawal of treatment and overdid it by feeling it had to call this point death. This would mean that the criteria were unnecessary at best and disingenuous at worst. But the medical records suggest that thresholds for discontinuation of care, and irreversible coma, were quite different.

For example, this new type of coma differed from other discontinuation cases and from other comas in the use of EEG. Of the total records reviewed, sixty-six (16 percent) had their treatment discontinued and seventy-one (17 percent) retrospectively met the Harvard criteria based on symptoms described in the record. These were not all the same cases, although those meeting the criteria were much more likely to have treatment ended. Of those who retrospectively met the criteria, twenty-seven (38 percent) had their treatment discontinued. Among the 352 who did not retrospectively meet the criteria, thirty-nine, or 11 percent, had notations indicating that their treatment was discontinued. I categorized the stated rationale in the record for deciding to discontinue care as either based on the EEG (even if other relevant findings were present), on the

EEG and other physical or laboratory findings, or only on other findings. Among those who met the criteria and had treatment discontinued, in nineteen cases (70 percent) the EEG was the reason specifically given for discontinuation, whereas it was the singular attributed reason in ten of the thirty-nine patients (26 percent) who had treatment discontinued but did not meet the Harvard criteria. So from this sampling, EEG increasingly became a benchmark for prognosis and ending of treatment in a general sense, but was also used much more frequently and specifically for those who would meet the criteria. While drawn from a convenience sample of records, this pattern suggests that features of these patients compelled a distinctly closer look at the "working brain" than did other patients for whom care was withheld. The criteria appear then to have captured and crossed more than a threshold for legitimate discontinuation or with-drawal of care in general, but captured a distinct condition and different kind of futility.

Of note, few cases of discontinuation of care involved discontinuation of respirators—only eleven patients across this decade from within this spe-cific sampling of those seen by Schwab's team and whose records were still accessible had a respirator turned off. While this is a very small subsample, it appears that hesitancy cut across cases meeting and not meeting the criteria, as six among the eleven retrospectively met criteria and five did not. It was resisted in patients for whom all other critical supportive care (e.g., vasopressors maintaining blood pressure) was discontinued. In these records, and in much of the literature reviewed herein, ending respirator care during this period seemed to be regarded as more of a commission than an omission, irrespective of condition. Consider, for example, one sixty-seven-year-old woman admitted to MGH in early 1963: She followed Fisher's step-by-step path toward a nonfunctioning brain, but that was not sufficient to stop treatment. This patient was "flaccid and quadroparetic and unresponsive to all but pain stimuli. Her eyes are fixed...Neither move to vigorous head turning. Both pupils...react very weakly to light. Seems quite certain she has coned. I doubt process is reversible at this time." Things soon further deteriorated: "The present situation seems almost hopeless: although her pupils...still respond to light, she is quite unresponsive with flaccid paralysis, supported with respirator and with aramine in a precarious state." Hours later it was reported: "Pupils fixed, no calorics." Finally, "There was no BP or pulse palpable and ECG showed no activity and respirator was taken off the patient, who expired quietly @ 2:10 AM." After her heart stopped, the respirator was discontinued. But the physicians writing entries here noted that the patient "died" only after the respirator was discontinued. The visibility of the dead nervous system and even, in this case, a nonbeating heart, did not outshine the visible appearance of "breathing." This illustrates the distance to be filled for neurological signs to be adequate for considering a patient already dead, and underscores the power of the respirator and the respiring body in shaping the *experience* of omission versus commission. Even decades later, routine use of brain death still involves declaring death first, then removing the respirator, as it did here and in other medical records where death was declared after irreversible cardiac arrest. At this time at MGH, in these records, respirators (as opposed to ending other life supporting treatment) usually were turned off after death. So in fashioning criteria, Schwab and the Committee were describing an equivalent to the end of heartbeat, a set of circumstances on par with respirator discontinuation as a marker of death itself. Brain death, to those who developed the criteria for it, emerges less as a proxy term for permission to withhold care than as an imperative for doing so. Reading through these cases reinforces this impression.

SIGNALS AND SIGNS

In 1959, near the outset of this decade of activity, one man entered the hospital with multiple worsening problems: likely renal failure, heart failure, and "dilated fixed pupils, centrally fixed eyes." His continued capability for "breathing in gasps" reflected some preserved brain function, but the signs pointed to his being "terminal from combined organ failure...Cannot forseeably [sic] reverse these multiple disorders. Supportive care." Although vague and often fragmented, descriptions like this one of the neurologic features of these "multiple disorders" determined the gap between aggressive treatment and "supportive care." One patient had mixed intact cranial reflexes (some absent, some present) and was responsive to pain, but had no vertical eye movements. He was described as "alert, able to blink" but showed enough impairment to qualify as "unresponsive" long enough to discourage significant treatment: "plan has been *not to treat other than for his comfort*, in view of age plus 8 weeks of unresponsiveness." The vague and varying barometer of neurologic status in these accounts was enough to shape therapeutic imperatives. The chart of one patient, in September 1962, contains this dire assessment: "Waiting to see if neurological function returns will continue and make it wise to proceed with 4+ push to solve his other difficulties if possible." Later, "Pt somewhat more obtunded this evening—Prognosis still poor—will not add antibiotics." Over the next two days the patient however was "a bit lighter" and "continues to brighten up. Now talking a bit and showing much more movement in bed…in view of improvement begun on Pen. rx." However imprecise, neurologic status was increasingly relied upon for making decisions to limit care, whether or not it presented as irreversible coma. Commenting on the plight of a twenty-two-month-old child brought to MGH in October, 1962, a practitioner noted: "The general medical problems here seem to overshadow the basic neurological disturbance, however, the bulging extruding brain will probably supply the prognosis."

The conditions of death before dying elevated the visibility of neurologic signs, especially as prognostic signs. Neurologic criteria assumed, and required, greater precision because of this. In reading through the cases of patients at MGH whom Schwab and his colleagues together encountered, this process is visible—a gradual, fluctuating use of and comfort with a credible and reliable set of core signs that identified when a subset of these patients with irreversible consciousness were also in a state proximate to the full loss of bodily functioning.

Any effort to list the characteristics of irreversible coma that distinctly placed it beyond coma, beyond the moving neurological parts of the EEG research literature that supported consciousness and physiological survival, not surprisingly referred back to the EEG itself. The presumed objectivity, replicability and visibility of EEG seemed perfectly suited to meet this apparent need for greater precision of determining brain function and the consequences of neurological failure. EEG was referred to in the Harvard criteria as a "confirmatory" test. However, its role in actual decision making, at least in these patients at MGH—and especially in the composition and validation of the criteria—proved more important than that. The varying and evolving role of EEG helps describe how brain death seemed to make sense to Schwab, and to the physicians at MGH who requested EEGs from him.

This use of EEG to arbitrate standard work for severe coma evolved over time. For one thing, many cases cautioned drawing conclusions from EEG at the bedside. That caution is also ultimately reflected in the "whole brain" set of conditions and timelines in Schwab's "conservative guideline." For one thing, EEG could itself be misleading. In November of 1965 at MGH, a fifty-year-old woman with meningitis was found, in an EEG report penned by Schwab, to have had "no clear evidence of EEG activity... An EEG of 12/28 was flat, and one on 12/29 showed only very slight activity... Very little we can do... Almost certain she is terminal." But several weeks later, she "ma[de] copious spontaneous movements of all extremities," and left the hospital conversing, interacting, and moving all extremities. While not very common among the hundreds of cases reviewed, such turnarounds cautioned that other evidence was needed to declare death before dying.

A more common challenge was the ambiguity of the tracings themselves. A series of EEG readings tracking the condition of a pregnant patient with a barbiturate overdose in September of 1963 found first that "there is much muscle and movement artifact, but *very little real* brain activity here." Two days later, in the same patient, the "EEG shows *a little more* activity than the previous one... diffuse very low voltage fast and intermediate fast activity in all leads." Three days after that, "at regular gain, there is no EEG. No responses in EEG... NO *clear* EEG present." Another chart of a patient admitted to MGH that same year read: "EEG shows *almost* a complete absence of cortical activity in dominant hemisphere." In June, 1964, a man who became comatose after suffering an MI had an EEG showing "low voltage again of a very *questionable* sort. I am unwilling to say whether there is definite cerebral activity in this tracing…Markedly abnormal, *probably* no brain wave activity." Another 1964 report read: "EEG again is flat but shows bursts of 3–7/sec waves that I cannot explain." Later that day, a note in the chart interpreted this report to mean that the "EEG today [was] still *essentially* flat." A repeat EEG was needed to clarify things: "This time, the curious theta activity is not seen…no evidence of cerebral activity." For a fifty-eight-year-old patient admitted unconscious after a fall in August of 1965, withdrawal from pain was the only sign of a working nervous system: "Will get EEG to check cortical activity." That report found literally mixed signals: "With normal gains there is almost no activity. With the gains up at maximum there is a little amount of fluctuant activity which *may be* cerebral activity…*Doubtful* evidence of cerebral activity" [all emphases mine]. Caveats with respect to "artifact" were common, as were characterizations of the presence of waveforms as "very little," then "a little more," "probably," "maybe," "questionable," "doubtful," or "almost" "real" brain activity.

In Schwab's EEG reports, ambiguity of interpretations as to when the brain no longer worked diminished over time. Precise prognoses from EEG output often came not from the EEG alone but from how it interacted with and reinforced key physical findings. For a sixty-seven-year-old man, a surgery in March 1964 turned into an unexpected emergency with severe brain anoxia. The EEG found "no normal EEG" but some activity. A suggested repeat EEG found that "it is slightly encouraging that the record wasn't flat but the evidence for severe brain damage is present nevertheless. Pt responds a little more today to various stimuli but the overall prognosis is very poor." An additional EEG found "further improvement but clinically patient remains unchanged." EEG and physical exam were tethered—shared direction and intensity reinforced each other. Schwab's criteria ended up being those that described the point at which the outer limits of nervous function, discernible by physical examination, coincided with the limits of EEG to capture deterioration—as they did with a three-year-old who came to MGH in February of 1966 showing clinical evidence of absent neurologic functioning:

EEG...shows no evidence of electrical activity originating in the brain—pupils stopped responding to light at 4:40 PM. Blood pressure barely obtainable, No urine formed since this morning. In view of these findings the mechanical respiration was discontinued at this time. Spontaneous respirations did not resume—heartbeat ceased at 5:35 PM and patient declared dead at this time.

Schwab's criteria for absence of function reflected his accumulating experience with patients and his response to colleagues' requests. This meant following the course and reliability of physical and electroencephalographic signals—their fluctuation one with the other—in order to identify the conditions under which absent EEG activity also reflected physical findings that made sense. In April 1967, neurological examination of a thirty-six-year-old with encephalitis found that "his neurological status is unchanged and it does not appear likely to be changed it at all—He will be on Bird [respirator] for forseeable future and so I agree we need tracheostomy—and will so arrange." An EEG found that "in between these jerks the record is usually flat although not always so but these artifacts appear to obscure anything else. Thus no true cortical activity can be recognized although the possibility of its existence is not excluded entirely." Days later, as the clinical condition pronounced itself more unambiguously, so did the EEG: "EEG shows no definite cortical activity. Situation is hopeless." This young patient died soon thereafter. On the other hand, early the following month, another patient with a dismal EEG record had this follow-up:

Repeat EEG today shows "remarkable recovery" from yesterday with evidence of some activity whereas there was complete absence yesterday....She is totally a-reflexic, bilateral upgoing toes, no response to noise or painful stimulus. Absent corneal reflexes, minimal pupillary reaction to light. No spontaneous respiration off the respirator. The situation continues to be extremely grim. In spite of improved EEG, it is still markedly diffusely abnormal.

Schwab's criteria for irreversible coma sought then to describe the coincident irreversible loss of sustainable physiology *and* the machinery of consciousness. The apparently objective, visible qualities of EEG, along with efforts to standardize the physical, neurological examination of coma, mutually reinforced each other for that purpose.

Disagreement about whether to emphasize brainstem versus "whole" brain (brainstem and cortex) signs in the criteria continued among neurologists long after the Report's publication. This was taken by commentators on brain death to be a sign that brain death was really a dispute over conceptual biases regarding whether death resulted from loss of "higher" consciousness and personhood on the one hand, versus loss of "lower" functions and biological integration on the other. Within the medical thought-style, for these physicians the debate between brainstem and whole brain positions was not a conceptual one but a technical one. Either position sought to capture a "whole" loss of higher and lower brain function. They differed over what parsimony of symptoms offered an acceptably accurate reading of those losses. Rather than a dispute over meanings or priority of mental versus biological aspects of personhood, these disagreements were about medical knowledge, about the sensitivity and specificity of certain outward physical signs to describe inward details, and the conditions and reasons for knowing them. In this way it was also a difference over how to understand the findings of Moruzzi and Magoun, and how that generation of research described in Chapter Four translated to the bedside—whether among its implications was that "an isolated cortex is useless to an animal."

Since at least 1955, MGH neurologist C. Miller Fisher had focused on these physical signs. Independent of Schwab, he developed a physical examination to determine what was happening in the brains of comatose, respirator-bound patients. Fisher recalled that as director of the Stroke Service at MGH, he began that year to try to identify physical characteristics that correlated with level of coma and that could be used to predict outcome: "We had to get into it...we had no language to describe them or rate them or anything...the examination of the sick [comatose] patient was chaotic."[26] Serial editions of Roy Grinker's *Neurology*, a prominent neurology textbook published from the 1930s through the 1960s, for example, included minimal descriptions of the examination of the comatose patient.[27] Fisher drew upon observations of brainstem and higher level function that appeared in the clinical literature, such as those involving maintenance of gaze upon rapid head movement (the oculocephalic reflex), or eye movements resulting from pouring iced water in a person's ears (caloric stimulation) and lightly touching the corneas (the corneal reflex), as well as responses to general motor reflex stimulation; he further considered how all these correlated with lesions at autopsy. Fisher recalled that by 1957, he was advising decisions to turn off respirators based on confidence in his exam to predict the irreversible loss of the central nervous structures' ability to maintain any cortical activity or independent vegetative functions. With few exceptions, families participated in these decisions with little fanfare or controversy.[28]

Fisher coined what later became commonplace names for neurological syndromes and terms; in particular, he established a nomenclature to describe brain hemorrhage and infarcts by combining careful patient observation and pathological correlation.[29] His examination of the comatose patient, not published in detail until 1969, reflects this kind of approach. It was an inventory of symptoms and a description of their functional and prognostic significance. Fine detail mattered in order to accurately describe the nature and location of the coma's cause. "Athetoid restlessness," "rhythmic myoclonus," "fishmouthing (dropping of the lower jaw at inspiration)," and "ocular bobbing" all were often missed or poorly understood signs that could provide diagnostic information above and beyond the more traditional examination of pupillary light response, reflexes, respirations, and response to pain and other stimuli. Fisher detailed the value of certain cranial nerve and brainstem reflexes, easily missed combinations of symptoms, or order of appearance of symptoms that revealed the neurological condition within.

Fisher described two general causes of coma: severe injury to the cerebral hemisphere, or "indirect functional paralysis of cortical function consequent upon inactivity of the ascending reticular activating system."[30] The latter might be captured through unique physical findings on examination. While Bremer, Magoun, Moruzzi, Penfield, and others "accumulated an extensive knowledge of the relation of alertness and consciousness to the functions of the brain stem...when human coma cases are discussed the details of the neurologic examination are almost totally lacking."[31] That examination had to focus on objective correlates of brainstem functioning: "Coma can be accurately defined only in terms of a complete neurological examination."[32] This relied on replicable physical findings, ones far more reliable than vague descriptions of awareness or consciousness: "Introduction of the terms conscious and unconscious has been avoided here, for these have to do with the content of 'psychic' experience, and although dependent upon 'alertness', alertness by no means insures full consciousness."[33] Fisher went on to explain these findings in greater detail:

> Recently it has been suggested that the death of a patient be defined in terms of an electroencephalogram, namely electrical silence or the absence of brain waves. Preferable to this method is a meticulous assessment by a neurologist skilled in the interpretation of comatose states and the recognition of extensive irreversible damage to the brain stem—cessation of all respiratory movements, fixed dilated pupils, fixed eyeballs in the central position, absent corneal reflexes and flaccid limbs. Since the introduction of modern respirators in 1955, we have followed the course of over 200 comatose patients with these signs and none with a structural non-metabolic insult to the brain has made any recovery despite vigorous supportive measures carried out for periods of up to three weeks. Lesser deficits may also be incompatible with useful recovery but such states are difficult to define.[34]

Fred Plum also felt that physical clues alone about the integrity of the brainstem were sufficient. In 1966 Plum published, with Jerome Posner, a still authoritative book on the examination of coma called *The Diagnosis of Stupor and Coma*; the second edition was published in 1972. The change in content across these two volumes reflects a change in the ways that observations of coma, along with work on EEG and arousal mechanisms, guided conclusions about the ends of treatment and the end of life.

The book, essentially an elaboration of a paper Plum published with Donald McNealy in 1962, laid out how Plum considered the steps leading to damage to the upper brainstem as the usual cause of coma.[35] In this book, Plum revisited the haunting decerebrate patients of Wilson, Cairn's cases of akinetic mutism, von Economo's experience with encephalitis, and a range of observations in the clinical literature of "pathological sleep" and sensory-motor signs in brainstem and third ventricle injuries.[36] He also reviewed well-described syndromes of supratentorial (above the brainstem structures) lesions, and patients for whom edema from cerebral anoxia and trauma also caused swelling and impingement on lower brain structures coincident with worsening responsiveness and nervous system function. Taken together, these cases led Plum to conclude that most roads to coma traveled through the brainstem. The work of Moruzzi, Magoun, and Lindsley on the RAS bolstered the view that these clinical signs should be interpreted to mean that the brainstem was the final common pathway to coma. Plum considered diagnosis of coma to be the task of distinguishing between (1) supratentorial lesions causing downward damage that eventually reached the brainstem; (2) direct brainstem lesions; (3) more unusual severe bilateral hemispheric injury that usually derived from metabolic and, in rare cases, from catastrophic anoxic injury; and (4) psychogenic causes. The book was organized around detailed descriptions of these four possibilities, and the clinical correlates that should alert the clinician to each.

The first edition of the book included research by Jouvet on the complex regulation of sleep, along with Lindsleys's musings on the RAS and thalamic reticular systems as the mechanism of true consciousness defined as selective attention and sensory ordering. Plum focused on the argument that coma usually meant brainstem damage and was generally different from the clouding of consciousness found in cortical damage. Exceptions to this rule were easy to identify—barbiturate or anesthesia use, or massive bilateral cortical damage. Plum was more circumspect in following through on the implications of this shift in focus from cortical to brainstem damage as the core cause of coma in terms of what it meant for drawing conclusions about irreversible coma. While helpful, EEG work on the brainstem was not definitive in this regard. Magoun, Plum would later point out, was talking about the RAS and EEG *waveforms*, not necessarily *consciousness*: "All consciousness requires arousal but all unconsciousness is not the absence of arousal. This was still a hard concept, even in the 1960s."[37] The irreversibly and completely unconscious body did not directly translate into the *cerveau isole*, at least not generally in the US experience at this time. Again, Bard's response to Magoun—that it may be impossible to know what a decerebrate animal experiences—remained quite relevant. The debate over brainstem approaches versus whole brain approaches (usually meaning loss of cortical EEG as well as loss of brainstem signs and greater rigor about absence of certain signs such as peripheral reflexes) would distinguish efforts in the United States from those in Britain to establish criteria for brain death, and capture the continued relevance of Magoun's question.[38]

But Plum and Posner's second edition showed more confidence in asserting that brainstem damage was the basis for coma and, then further, that if the brainstem were no longer functional, this provided enough certainty as to irreversible loss of the capacity for consciousness and related cortical activity. Significant research supporting that conclusion, even though published before the first edition appeared, was only included in this second edition. This work was cited to bolster the primary role of the brainstem in coma and to address more directly how loss of brainstem structures reliably meant the loss of consciousness. The second edition also elaborated more on describing RAS, this time including transcriptions of the 1958 symposium that had been edited by Jasper to summarize work on the reticular formation.[39] Plum described consciousness as "awareness of self and environment" and coma as "unarousable unresponsiveness." He endorsed the British Medical Research Council definition of coma as the "absence...[of] psychologically understandable response to external stimulus or inner need," which was similar to the phraseology that Adams added to the Report.[40] While Plum assigned to the brainstem and cortex the roles of maintaining conscious arousal and content, respectively, he agreed that there was enough evidence to say that both ultimately relied on brainstem functions. Therefore this edition more firmly indicated that loss of those functions meant irreversible loss of consciousness, irrespective of how the cortex was doing. He also included Mollaret and Goulon's paper coining "coma dépassé," and work on the pathology of brains of respirator-bound, comatose patients—all of which were not included in the 1966 edition. The very same citations of work by Moruzzi and Jouvet on the mechanisms of sleep in the first edition were used in the second to draw a different conclusion, reflecting the difference these interim years made. In the first edition, these citations supported vague acknowledgements that coma and sleep mechanisms might overlap. In the second edition, Plum is comfortable enough in his conclusions about the brainstem to use these same references to justify the conclusion that their mechanisms were in fact quite different.

In the space of five or six years, Plum became more secure in describing the prominence of the brainstem for coma, a transition he explicitly recognized.[41] This confidence was critical for a new section appearing in the second edition of *Diagnosis* to address a subject unremarked upon in the first: the subject, that is, of which signs constituted an irreversible coma indicating nonsurvival and perpetual unconsciousness.

In Plum's reading of the literature and his experience with patients, if examination found a nonfunctioning brainstem by reviewing the reflexes and responses served by that structure, then EEGs were unnecessary to determine irreversible coma. He felt Beecher and his Committee were too conservative. Similarly, preservation of some primitive stretch and postural reflexes unrelated to brainstem integrity did not exclude the diagnosis. His own criteria thus included total unawareness, lack of purposeful response to stimuli, and absence of brainstem function—that is, no spontaneous breathing or apnea, unreactive pupils, and absent oculocephalic and oculovestibular reflexes. These basically "British" brainstem criteria were still markedly similar to the whole-brain Harvard criteria. The latter was differentiated by a broader exclusion of peripheral reflexes (though also contingent upon them), as well as by reference to EEG and confirmatory testing to more completely avoid having to answer Magoun's question.

Over the next decades, these differences in criteria would narrow due to the accumulating—though still disputed—evidence of the redundancy of these confirmatory tests.

The whole-brain direction of the Committee not only reflected more caution as to whether some surviving cortex in the context of irreversibly nonfunctioning brainstem was relevant for consciousness. It also turned on the degree to which these signs described physiological survivability as well. For Schwab, and the Report, Plum's conclusions about permanent unconsciousness were necessary but not sufficient for a neurologically based finding of death—and also not fully conclusive.

THE BRAIN AND THE BODY

Reliable signs of the absence of capacity for consciousness were necessary but not sufficient to consider irreversible coma as a pronouncement. Regardless of whether one would argue that consciousness was the sine qua non of life and personhood, it could not be argued that a dead person could still have the capability for consciousness—one could not be considered dead if one were conscious. The neurologically empty body described by the criteria was one that, in this context of care and other physical signs, appeared to show itself to be physiologically empty as well, such that Schwab in his medical record notes began distinguishing the "cerebral" or "cortical" death from the "clinical" and "physiological" death of the irreversible coma patient.

For a patient seen in November 1958 with significant unresponsiveness to pain, but signs of continued brain and cranial nerve functioning, it was suggested that a "special EEG [be done] today to see what state of consciousness" the patient maintained. However, the "EEG [was] not contributory as hoped it might be." In the cases Schwab's EEG team was asked to see at MGH, "special" EEGs would become less special and more common guides for what they described, not only about the survivability of consciousness but also about overall physiological functioning. In May of 1959, a patient with pneumonia had a neurological examination generally consistent with what would become the Harvard criteria, save for the per-sistence, albeit poor, of spontaneous breathing. The record indicated that "the presumable amount of brainstem involvement is probably not revers-ible" and several days later noted: "on optimum antibiotics—appears jig is up. Cannot survive long." The following entry reported that the "Pt. died a respiratory death at 11:41 PM." No EEG was obtained, and in this case the interest in brainstem functioning arose, but in order to understand the likelihood of continued breathing. There is clear evidence in these records of a working understanding of the role of the brainstem in maintaining consciousness. Indeed, In March of 1962, Schwab's colleague Hannibal Hamlin suggested pushing the degree to which RAS integrity mattered, and could even manipulated, when he wrote the following about a patient:

Coma seems fairly deep—probably due to RAS depression...Can brainstem be stimulated to improve state of awareness by external EST [electric stimulation]...Would doubt it because of other factors assoc with or contributing to RAS suppression. But if EEG is not too disorganized...EST could be tried...If no response—brainstem damage might be considered irreversible.

EST as a means toward stimulating more direct repair of injured brainstem was not a successful strategy (though there have been intermittent efforts to revive interest in that possibility since). But as with the case described above where mention of the brainstem was in the context of assessing the status of respiratory function, not consciousness, these records tended less commonly or directly to focus specifically on the condition of the brainstem.

The pattern, at least in these records with disproportionate use of EEG among those who would retrospectively meet criteria seems to reflect a belief that redundant and more direct and visible validation of cortical loss was necessary. But, again, only part of the work brain death criteria had to do was to validate irreversible loss of consciousness. The whole-brain, as opposed to brainstem, direction of the Harvard criteria also reflected a response to inconsistency in the degree that this loss of cortical activity alone also captured central nervous system and overall functional loss more generally.

One forty seventy-one-year-old patient on Fisher's Stroke Service in February of 1961 showed significant unresponsiveness, but still had some rotation on one limb in response to pain and symmetrical reflexes. However, one physician noted "no cortical activity by EEG," and another that "the situation seems entirely hopeless." Orders were made to "D/C aramine streptomycin penicillin" to maintain the patient's blood pressure. In another situation in April 1962, a patient after a cardiac arrest was felt to need "no additional therapeutic suggestions. No heroics are indicated for indefinite cardiac maintenance." The medical record a few days later reinforced the physician's initial stance: "I really do not know if we have to continue the situation. The anoxic brain damage seems quite [unreadable]." But others noted: "He is making swallowing movements but does not direct gaze toward spoken voice." Nonetheless, "The EEG report is very close to being a pronouncement of no activity. Under the circumstances the prognosis is probably hopeless and should discourage anything except palliative [treatment]." At this point, medications supporting the patient's blood pressure were removed. These cases showed ambiguous signs of continued physical responsivity in light of evidence of irreversible loss of consciousness, and would not have met the Report's criteria. They illustrate both the degree to which brain function factored into decisions to determine and discontinue futile care, as well as the degree to which the eventual brain death criteria, in contrast and on purpose, went beyond that threshold to describe those who showed a further state of physiological failure.

Schwab established a routine that included the use of EEG to validate this state—first, a finding of a total lack of neurological responsiveness by exam; then a flat EEG, confirmed by a second; followed by withdrawal of treatment. Completely unresponsive except for spinal reflexes, a five-year-old girl had an EEG in February of 1965. The record showed that "after discussing findings with the parents, the mother requested that the Byrd machine be turned off. This was done as requested since there was no activity of EEG record." A twenty-five-year-old head injury victim was admitted that same month in "flaccid, areflexic" condition, with "pupils fixed and dilated." The record further noted that "pt may be candidate for EEG determination if there is any CNS function." That "determination" found "no EEG seen any leads any time in spite of increased gains. Probably cerebral death. Repeat in 24 hours if desired." The notes went on to say that the "EEG yesterday thought to show cortical death by Dr Schwab. Repeat today. I should think we should refrain from further transfusions, etc. Family aware of the situation." Another patient who fit this pattern was a fifty-nine-year-old man, admitted in May of 1966, who had stopped breathing. He met what would become the Harvard criteria: fixed pupils, no responsiveness or reflexes, and no breathing. The EEG was reported by Schwab as "essentially flat with no recognizable EEG. Should be repeated in 24 hours." That same day the chart read: "The EEG as reported by Dr. R. Schwab was 'no evidence of cortical activity.' After discussion between Mr. B and Dr. S it was Mr. B's decision to omit aramine fom IV's. The full implications of this were explained to Mr. B."

Consistent correlation between the tangible, flat EEG and the physical signs, nonsurvival, and irreversible loss of consciousness was reported in a series of three studies published from 1963 to 1968 in which Schwab worked to elaborate and, most significantly, confirm the prognostic value of his criteria. First with a series of ten patients, and finally with a large series of ninety cases with autopsy correlations, he felt he showed that his triad of clinical findings reliably indicated a dead brain *and* nonsurvival.[42] The first study, presented in 1962 and published in 1963, summarized a series of ten cases over the prior two years. These cases showed no spontaneous respiration or pupillary reflexes, absence of EEG, and no response to noxious stimuli (i.e., no heart rate change with eyeball pressure). This triad predicted brief survival and led Schwab to conclude that "in spite of cardiac actions, the patient is dead." Based on experience presented the following year with thirty-five more patients, Schwab likely was spurred to lengthen the time of isoelectric EEG to a twenty-four hour minimum between readings, a length that appeared in subsequent versions of his triad.[43]

In 1965, Schwab published a study of what he described as all of the cardiac or respiratory arrest patients on whom EEGs were performed at MGH. In those with flat EEG records, or records with markedly depressed voltage, death occurred in all cases with no interval of a return of consciousness.[44] Finally, in 1968, Schwab reported a series of ninety patients who met his now condensed "triad" of criteria for "irreversible coma": no reflexes, no spontaneous respirations, and an isoelectric EEG. This triad correlated with marked necrosis of brain tissue at autopsy. The criteria predicted nonsurvival as well as destruction of brain tissue. The Harvard Report emerged from this mixture of reliable, brainstem-based but cortical EEG-confirmed signs of a lost capability for consciousness, which also indicated nonsurvival. The Report summarized irreversible coma as the "Complete absence of receptivity of all forms of sensory stimulation and a lack of response to stimuli and inner need." This unresponsiveness "always [had] coincident paralysis of the brainstem and basal ganglionic mechanisms." Brainstem loss, up through the thalamus, was the physical finding correlating with loss of "response to … inner need." By specifying in this "summary" section that brainstem pathology was at the root of irreversible coma, the Report aimed to distinguish spurious spinal reflexes from relevant responses—a point the "British" view underscored. Why, then, didn't the criteria simply and directly adopt Plum's eventual confidence in the brainstem?

To start, for Adams, work on RAS—the "diencephalic regulator"—still fell short of a completely satisfying account of consciousness.[45] Conditions like akinetic mutism left unsettled the nature of the brainstem and consciousness. Adams recalled Committee discussions of syndromes such as akinetic mutism and what would come to be called *persistent vegetative state*. These were syndromes against which the Committee needed to set boundaries. They were not ready to judge these as markers of "higher" death of the brain or person—not because of a starting point of philosophical commitments, but because of limited confidence in what these clinical syndromes reflected physiologically and functionally, and lack of reliable terminology with which they could be described.

Knowledge about the "diencephalic regulator" lent confidence, but also the expectation that the scope of the criteria described the lack of a "waking" brain as well as the absence of a "working" brain and body. Based on comments by William Sweet, the "summary" section likely emerged out of debates between Sweet, Adams, and Schwab around how completely physical signs of brainstem dysfunction alone described irreversible coma and death. Why suggest a confirmatory EEG? Why require (and then later seem to backtrack on) absent spinal reflexes and all movement? Sweet recalls taking the British view that all that was needed was clinical evidence of no brainstem, which primarily included apnea, absent cranial reflexes, and unresponsivity. But the other three "beat on me," and remained concerned about whether evidence was indeed adequate that there would be no recovery of consciousness if there were remnants of EEG activity (e.g., nests of cells in the cortex) as the British view could allow. Sweet felt the more restrictive view of the Report would "hold up" transplantation.[46] Adams, though, proved decisive. He cited the line of research, beginning with Moruzzi, Magoun, Dempsy, and Morison, which established that the regulator of consciousness was in a small part of the brainstem. But, as with Sweet's recollection, Adams also was mindful that for the purposes of describing a coma that pronounced death, the data (such as Schwab's) that more reliably demonstrated not just irreversible unconsciousness but nonsurvivability pointed to broader criteria.

Practice at MGH relied upon this mutual reinforcement of EEG and physical findings in ultimately describing the features of the brain dead condition. Beecher's confidence in Schwab's triad, both at Eliasburg and in drafting the Report, rested to a large degree on his experience at MGH (and the growing practice in other centers) of including isolelectric EEG as a criterion. Almost eighteen months after the Report appeared, Beecher gave advice to a Johns Hopkins surgeon—who was also leading an effort in Maryland to establish guidelines for brain death—reiterating the importance of EEGs within Schwab's timeframe and emphasizing that data did not yet support a change in practice.[47] Adams' edits to the criteria positioning EEG as a fourth and conditional criteria don't seem, then, to have been intended to diminish EEG use, but more likely to underscore, as he later put it, that "the point of the article was that you could circulate with no brain and that society should recognize that to be without a brain was more equivalent to death then stopping of the heart."[48] Eventually, though, additional data and clinical consensus would move more toward agreement on a limited need for EEG and on Adam's highlighting the loss of receptivity and response to inner need as key to what the criteria described.

The still tentative connection between what was known from research, and what was found with patients, called for more conservative criteria, in the view of the Committee—especially as a basis for the standardization of a condition that pronounced death. Schwab was explicitly asked if his criteria established "death" of the "higher" or "lower" centers, or both. Schwab replied that the criteria established both, but attributed this to the loss of the "lower centers," which Sugar and Gerard,[49] his most cited source, showed had the longest survival times among brain regions in the face of anoxia. If the lower centers were dead, "one can certainly assume that the higher centers are also dead."[50] But to *know* that from the outside required findings that might exceed simply testing brainstem integrity.

This was further underscored by cases where it seemed that brainstem function remained but cortical function apparently did not. In 1963, for example, a fifty-year-old man was unresponsive with absence of most midbrain and brainstem findings, such as response to pain, pupillary reflexes, and other cranial, ocular, and auditory nerve reflexes. But on exam, he had some residual lower brainstem reflexes, including slight gag and tongue reflexes, and the record noted this activity:

> [The patient was] showing functions of the lower pons and medulla but little evidence of function of any higher level of nervous activity. The prognosis is extremely poor and there is little to suggest that the most major therapeutic efforts would result in significant patient salvage. An EEG would be of aid in evaluating level of cerebral cortical damage. [That] EEG shows no electrical activity (completely flat record) over 20 minutes of recording. In our experience this would indicate that the prognosis for recovery is *nil*.

So some cases suggested that when it came to survival, irreversible cortical loss, may have been a more sensitive sign. Reinforcing this learned need to

trust but verify the consequences of lost brainstem function, and to distinguish cortical death from just grave prognosis, one physician caring for a
patient with coma in January of 1966 noted that an "EEG repeated today
again fails to show any evidence of cortical activity. Imp—There is no clinical or electrical evidence of function of the cerebral cortex *despite continuing brain stem activity*. The likelihood of a return of cerebral function to
anywhere near a normal state in this patient is now very small" [emphasis
mine]. This conclusion was explained by Young: "[EEG] is as flat a record
as I have seen, implying widespread cerebral death. This is not the picture
following brainstem infarction (cortex remains electrically active with diffuse slow waves)...Therefore I think we have to ascribe deep coma [with-
out] any reflexes except [decreased] plantars to widespread brain damage
following cardiac and/or respiratory arrest." Similarly, there was risk of
EEG overdetermining complete loss of cortical activity as the gold standard endpoint. In another patient with a flat EEG, seen in December 1967,
the EEG report conveyed that "it is obvious that there is some cerebral
activity still present in view of the brisk pupillary response. It would be
reasonable to carry on with present regime of Rx." There often appeared a
preference for cortical functioning or reliable evidence of its loss in making prognoses more generally, a kind of anti-British view: "Prognosis is
dismal in view of EEG and physical status....No corneals, no EOM on
Doll's head, no pupillary reaction with pupils...Flaccid, no DTR's, no
reaction to painful stimuli." That said, another note read: "She still mani-
fests a few brainstem reflexes, *but the important fact here is that the cerebral hemispheres are essentially dead*. Please do not order any chemistries
or other diagnostic tests" [emphasis mine].

Whole, cortical, and brainstem-only signs were complexly distinguished and sorted. The "beating up" Sweet described by Schwab and
Adams makes sense in the context of these cases. If there was to be a
standard practice, it would be better to err on more sensitive, rather than
specific, criteria. In these cases at MGH where Schwab's team was asked
for EEG consultation, physicians making decisions showed this preference for the collection of signs that the whole brain was absent activity by
reading the cortex. As quoted above, Schwab increasingly used the term

"cortical death" as the ultimately important factor in either EEG tracings (which measured activity of the cortex) or physical neurological examination. Remarking on the case of one unfortunate fifteen-year-old, who was injured in a motor vehicle accident in April of 1967 and who met what would be the Harvard criteria as well, Schwab wrote that despite the lack of the physical examination findings at the core of those criteria, ultimately there was "no evidence of electrical activity... This is compatible with cortical death... There is no evidence of cortical electrical activity in this study." A few months before the Report came out, Schwab's lab reported on the EEG of a forty-four-year-old woman: "There is no EEG in this record... this second flat EEG, 48 hrs after the first, means that there is no chance of cortical recovery." A fifty-one-year-old man treated in 1964 for a cardiac arrest after withdrawal from alcohol was described as "a desperate situation where there seem to be too many strikes against the patient to consider survival possible. At this point I would give no further pressor agents but treat symptomatically, continuing respirator and IV fluids, until heart action stops." A subsequent EEG was read by Schwab to show "no EKG or EEG seen; patient clinically, as well as physiologically, dead." The relevance of cortical loss as the measure of *coma dépassé* depended on the other legs of the triad that reinforced the connection between irreversible loss of consciousness (through redundant signs of brainstem failure) and overall physiological failure. Read another record in 1966:

> The pt's upper brainstem (midbrain) was functionally transected in the EW as shown by fixed dilated pupils s globe movement to doll's head or ice water calorics—now the medulla is failing as shown by absent spontaneous respirations and now falling BP. Would favor EEG today and in 24 hrs if pt 'lives' that long—anticipate both will be flat.

Schwab's evolving phraseology reflected this experienced redundancy of cardiac standstill as a marker for *physiological* death when what he called *clinical* death, in terms of irreversible cortical and brainstem failure, were found. Summarizing the condition of a two-year-old patient, in coma after a fall and subsequent cardiac arrest and admitted in December of 1966, one physician noted the situation this way: "EEG x 2 with no cort. activity demonstrable makes any statement about heart, etc. academic." The EEG report captured the concurrent "deaths" that were visible and managed in this world of death before dying: "Recording on a *deceased pt* is abnormal because of absence of all electrical activity…This is clinical death." (emphasis mine). Of another patient cared for after a stroke in October 1966, a physician wrote: "I suspect we could keep cardiorespiratory system functioning for an indeterminate period, but with no cerebral activity there is little rational reason for doing so." Reliance on cortical death, understood as a reinforcement of brainstem death, became more routine and explicit in the records of cases Schwab's team was called to see for EEG. In July of 1967, one of Fisher's former Fellows wrote the following report for an eighteen-year-old who sustained head trauma after a car accident and met the full set of the Harvard criteria:

> I have discussed in detail with Mr. and Mrs. C—about the significance of the EEG with absent brain waves; they understand fully that his respirations are being controlled completely and that his heart continues to function because of respiratory assistance. They have agreed that if additional EEG shows no electrical activity that the respirator be discontinued.

NEW NORMS, NEW KNOWLEDGE

These MGH records also show the contradictions and ambivalence that came with more technologically intensive medicine and that appeared long before, and continued through and presumably long after, the appearance of brain death. In 1958, about when Schwab began cataloguing cases, the record for a patient with massive, terminal, internal bleeding documents that she was regularly "begging to be allowed to die pain free. Further attempts at transfusion not carried out." Yet when found with no heartbeat, the patient underwent tracheal suction, chest compressions, and intracardiac injections of epinephrine. A year later, a physician's note about whether to change a breathing tube of his six-year-old comatose patient as a precaution against future infection reflects much of the back and forth around the calculus of omissions and therapeutics in end of life decision making that was just emerging medicine at this time: "Of course she will probably not survive long enough for…tracheal inflammation to become apparent—but as long as we are making an attempt it seems worthwhile to make it in such a way that it won't be self-defeating if by remote chance it should be successful." In 1962, as Schwab's EEG lab linked his triad of symptoms (the lack of any reflexes, spontaneous breathing, or EEG) to nonsurvival, his team consulted on a patient without evidence of any brainstem function as tested via examination of the cranial nerves: "No EOM, no corneal, no facial grimace, no gag. No DTR's, no response plantars flaccid. No response to pain…EEG still flat this AM…Beyond maintaining her cardiorespiratory function to some extent, there is no evidence of viable CNS at this time." However, when her heart stopped, vigorous efforts were still made to revive her.

These medical records show repeated cases in which caregivers identified and agreed with the criteria and what they meant, but aggressively treated patients even when the heart stopped. Just a year before the Report appeared, a woman with cardiac arrest had an "official EEG report [which] has been read as no activity and will be repeated tomorrow." The next day, the patient "remain[ed] hypotensive on levophed without detectable CNS activity on 2nd EEG." But when she had another cardiac arrest, she was aggressively treated with multiple cardiac shocks and epinephrine injections. In 1966, another unfortunate patient, who was comatose, had a recording that was "grossly abnormal because of absence of electrical activity…This is compatible with clinical death." A same-day confirmatory EEG found "no change…Findings still are those of clinical death." And yet, aggressive treatment continued.

Beecher's goal, in part, was to make a new effective standard, or set of standards, in this context. Robert Young, Schwab's Fellow, observed that a prominent tension in the Committee meetings he attended arose over whether individual clinicians—considering their knowledge of pathology and familiarity with Fisher's experience—could diagnose irreversible coma based on their "judgment" alone. Likely as a result of seeing mixed and unpredictable practices and applications of available examination methods, Beecher and Schwab argued for standardization of criteria.[51] About the time Beecher moved to form the Committee, some signs of standardization appeared. One note confidently and crisply surmised that a forty-year-old comatose man admitted in October of 1967 had an "EEG x 2 absent reflexes for legal death." And earlier that year, a new term appeared in these medical records: "I see absolutely no chance of any recovery whatsoever and pronounce the *brain dead*. With husband's consent I recommend turning off mechanical aids and declaring pt dead" [emphasis mine]. The patient met the eventual Harvard criteria of no cranial reflexes, responsiveness, or ability to breathe. After describing that examination, a note appears in the record written by the patient's husband: "I authorize the termination of automatic artificial respiration on my wife."

The relationship between the brain's death and physiological dissolution was more an evolving finding than a principled position. Bioethics critics would argue that in reality, however, the brain death criteria outlined by the Report did, at least implicitly, adopt a conceptual position of life as biological integration, and of the brain as the integrator-in-chief. That position, it was argued, became more untenable as life support methods improved. For Beecher, and it appears similarly so for many working at the bedsides at MGH, any such position was an endpoint, not a starting point. Dis-integration did not have to be proven to be a legitimate guiding concept. It was a lived reality and target on the wards at MGH and elsewhere. If ICU technology has changed the way disintegration is understood since the criteria appeared, it has done so through changes in how to prove, describe, make visible and test things in the medical context, and the purposes that driven them. *Those* changes deserve our deep understanding, rather than the conceptual labels that may describe those changes. Preoccupation with the latter labels rather than the former knowledge practices would prove to have substantial consequences, as discussed in the next chapter, for example in changes to how death was seen as necessary before removing organs for transplant.

The Harvard criteria described (as any death criteria should) how the longstanding distinction between omission and commission at the heart of guiding medical action become so thinly separated as to have no meaning in practice. If commission (intensive care on a neurologically empty body) was unethical experiment, then its omission was not an act of removal but recognition of what was so: that death was present before dying. These touchstones of medical action and experimentation were not defined through discursive, conceptual, analysis and debate, but through pragmatic use, accumulated evidence, and comparative experience with death and dying in the medical context.

Taking on these meanings not from some external conceptual perspective, but from the perspective of how meanings pragmatically worked in practice through use of inter-observable facts between participants, leaves us facing larger questions about the consequences of choosing to heal bodies through manipulation of biological mechanisms. What are the tools for generating, verifying, and living with the sorts of knowledge needed to do that? How much are these constrained by the body, or instead open to our own ends, such that this knowledge serves goals we value? These questions invite taking seriously the ontology of medicine; the ways that scientific methods of verification, however imperfect, unavoidably shape reality and broker values. They also acknowledge the constraints that raises for hard choices that ethical analysis, explored in the following chapter as applied to brain death, could neither solve nor remove.

Medical knowledge and action indeed shape the messy tangle we carry on with our biological selves and what we consider human nature to be. That knowledge and action has to be deeply engaged. Beecher's pragmatic response and description of how that knowledge works, and has to work, as a starting point for addressing these dilemmas, was a substantive one. Histories have instead generally consigned Beecher and the Report, to a role in justifying the bioethics narrative, which he, and the events described in this book, challenged.

NOTES

1. Robert Young, who succeeded Schwab as director of the Brain Wave Laboratory at MGH, confidently claimed first status in an obituary in the *Archives of Neurology*. See "Robert S. Schwab, M.D.," *Archives of Neurology* 27 (September, 1972): 271–72. Schwab's primary research assistant at the lab, John Barlow, eulogized Schwab as well, with the more qualified "one of the first" claims in "Obituary," *Journal of the Neurological Sciences* 19 (1973): 257–58. Most of the literature that I have come across describing Schwab's life and/or development of EEG echoes Young's version.

2. Alan Rubinstein, "And she's not only merely dead, she's really most sincerely dead," Letters, *The Hastings Center Report* 39, no. 5 (September–October 2009): 4–5.

3. I rely on surviving copies of the draft that belonged to Schwab and Murray throughout this study and thus may not specify which version when quoted, unless specific marginalia or source of edit evidence is unclear. They can be found respectively in Box 6, Folders 23 and 21, Beecher Papers. The same is true for the other versions. Changes resulting in and to the June 3 and June 7 draft are primarily from Beecher's copies, which can be found in Box 6, Folders 32 and 33, Beecher Papers. Adams' copies also contain other confirmation attributing edits to him (as do notes on Beecher's copies) in Box 6, Folder 18. June 13 version edits rely upon Beecher's versions in Folder 33 and Adams' versions in Folder 18. Unless specifying a particular issue, I will not cite these sources again below.

4. Box 6, Folder 23, Beecher Papers.

5. Box 6, Folder 36, Beecher Papers.

6. J. F. Alderete, F. R. Jeri, E. P. Richardson Jr., S. Sament, R. S. Schwab, and R. R. Young, "Irreversible coma: a clinical electroencephalographic and neuropathological study," *Transactions of the American Neurological Association* 93 (1968): 16–20. He similarly wrote to Beecher in comments on the April 11 draft that ending care for those with irreversible comas will "allow the heart to stop which is the moment of death." Schwab to Beecher, Box 6, Folder 23, Beecher Papers.

7. Schwab to Beecher, Folder 23, Beecher Papers.

8. Schwab to Beecher, Folder 23, Beecher Papers.

9. Robert Schwab, Memorandum, "American EEG Society Committee on Problem of Cerebral Death," Box 6, Folder 36, Beecher Papers.

10. Beecher's copy of June 3, 1968 draft, Box 6, Folder 32, Beecher Papers.

11. H. H. Bendixen et al., *Respiratory Care* (St. Louis: CV Mosby Co., 1965), 4.

12. See Henning Pontoppidan, "The development of respiratory care and the Respiratory Intensive Care Unit (RICU): a written oral history," in *"This is no humbug!" Reminiscences of the Department of Anesthesiology at the Massachusetts General Hospital*, ed. Richard J. Kitzler (Boston: MGH), 151–77; and Pontoppiden, interview with the author.

13. Schwab, "Manuscript outline for book proposal, 'Medico-Legal Aspects of Cerebral Death.'"

14. Hannibal Hamlin, "Life or death by EEG," *JAMA* 190, no.2 (October 12, 1964): 120–22, 120.

15. R. S. Schwab, F. Potts, and A. Bonazzi, "EEG as an aid in determining death in the presence of cardiac activity (ethical, legal and medical aspects)," *EEG and Clinical Neurophysiology* 15 (1963): 147–48. See also "Criteria to determine death are based on data from EEG," *Medical Tribune*, July 9, 1962, 1, 22. An accompanying editorial remarked how modern medicine is challenging distinctions between life and death, as well as the reliability of signs of cardiac function and respiration. Of note, no mention is made of transplantation.

16. "EEG termed guide to resuscitation," *Medical Tribune*, November 8, 1963, 1, 27.

17. Hannibal Hamlin, "Life or death by EEG," *JAMA* (October 12, 1964): 120–22, 121–22.

18. William Sweet, interview with the author, September 9, 1991.

19. Earl Ubell, "Death Defined," *New York Herald Tribune*, Sunday, February 14, 1965. See also a Boston newspaper account of Hamlin's address before the American Medical Association that informed the *JAMA* paper: Loretta McLaughlin, "Brain Waves Sign of Life," *Boston Herald-Traveler,* 1964. In both of these newspaper accounts and in other press coverage of this work at MGH, no connection to transplant is made by Hamlin, Schwab, or the authors.

20. R. S. Schwab, F. Potts, and A. Bonazzi, "EEG as an aid in determining death in the presence of cardiac activity (ethical, legal and medical aspects)," *Electroencephalography and Clinical Neurophysiology* 15 (1963): 147–48, 147.

21. See letter from Rosoff's secreatry to Schwab, Ocotober 31, 1968, copied from Rosoff's personal papers and used with his permission. The Soviet conference is in itself of interest. Negovsky, some of whose work was translated in the West, invited Schwab and directed a large institute devoted to "reanimation" utilizing a range of techniques, such as transfusing super-oxygenated blood. A wide range of work was resented by the Soviets focusing on how to prolong and revive the presumably comatose and brain-injured. However, they were very interested in how to prognosticate recovery of brain functioning. See G. Pampiglione, "A Report on the Symposium on Recovery after Resuscitation Moscow, November 1968," manuscript copy, Joan Schwab Papers; and Robert Schwab, "Report on the 5-Day Symposium on Recovery Period After Resuscitation Pathophysiology and Treatment in Experiment and Clinics," manuscript copy, Joan Schwab Papers. Schwab presented the triad as submitted to the Ad Hoc Committee. The papers were published as *Vostanoveetyelnee Peryod Posle Ozhyblyenya,* (or "The Recovery Period after Resuscitation") in 1970. See also V. A. Nogovsky, "Some physiopathologic regularities in the process of dying and resuscitation," *Circulation* 23 (March 1961): 452–57. Here, Negovsky made the point that life support interventions now were being applied to manage the process of dying. That process required a shift to assessing the state of the brain in order to assess the appropriateness of such interventions.

22. Sidney Rosoff, interview with the author, April 20, 1998.

23. "The EEG in Establishing Brain Death: A 10 Year Report with Criteria and Legal Safeguards in the 50 States," manuscript copy, Joan Schwab Papers. The copy states it was presented June 8, 1967, and that the criteria—now simplified to no hypothermia or anesthesia, "no reflexes or spontaneous breathing, or muscle activity, no

clinical or EEG response to noise or pitch" and repeatable "24 or 48 hours later"—
are notes to have "been fully approved by the authorities at the hospital, various
medial examiners in the area, two district attorneys, and the Medico-legal department at Harvard Medical School."

24. Fred Plum, interview with the author, April 20, 1998.
25. As described further below, Fisher was motivated by facing comatose patients
    in large numbers as the director of the new Stroke Service, which consolidated
    the examination and care of these patients. Henning Pontoppidan, who was the
    first director of Beecher's respiratory unit, credits the collection of such patients
    with the enhanced visibility of the problem of futility, as rare decisions by many
    practitioners segued into many such decisions by fewer specializing practitioners.
    Pontoppidan, interview with author, November 19, 1991.
26. C. Miller Fisher, interview with the author, August 30, 1991.
27. For example, see successive volumes through much of the twentieth century of Roy
    R. Grinker's text *Neurology*, published in serial editions in 1931, 1937, 1943, 1949,
    1960, and 1966.
28. C. Miller Fisher, interview with the author, December 6, 1996. Fisher's chronol-
    ogy of developing and using such an examination is corroborated by Fellows,
    who worked with him at this time. Vincent Perlo, interview with the author, July
    30, 1991.
29. For a brief summary, see Raymond D. Adams and Edward P. Richardson Jr., "Salute
    to C. Miller Fisher," *Archives of Neurology* 38 (March 1981): 137–39.
30. C. Miller Fisher, "The neurological examination of the comatose patient," *Acta
    Neurologica Scandinavica:* Supplementum 36, no. 45 (1969): 6.
31. Ibid., 5.
32. Ibid., 6.
33. Ibid., 10.
34. Ibid., 53–54.
35. Donald McNealy and Fred Plum, "Brainstem dysfunction with supratentorial mass
    lesions," *Archives of Neurology* 7 (July 1962): 26–48.
36. Prominent among these is a paper co-authored with Ray Adams on syndromes
    found with patients who had occlusions of the basilar artery, a main arterial supply
    to the brainstem. See Charles S. Kubik and Raymond D. Adams, "Occlusion of the
    basilar artery: a clinical and pathological study," *Brain* 69, no. 2 (June 1946): 6.
37. Fred Plum, interview with the author, April 20, 1998.
38. Eelco F. M. Wijdicks, "The transatlantic divide over brain death determination and
    the debate," *Brain* 135, no. 4 (2011): 1321–31.
39. Herbert Jasper et al., *Reticular Formation of the Brain* (Boston: Little, Brown and
    Company, 1958).
40. Plum and Posner, *Diagnosis of Stupor and Coma*, 2nd ed. (Philadelphia: FA Davis
    Company, 1972), 2, 5.
41. Plum, interview with the author, April 20, 1998.
42. R. S. Schwab, F. Potts, and A. Bonazzi, "EEG as an aid in determining death
    in the presence of cardiac activity (ethical, legal and medical aspects),"
    Electroencephalography and Clinical Neurophysiology 15 (1963): 147–48; Judith

Hockaday, Frances Potts, Eve Epstein, Anthony Bonazzi, and Robert S. Schwab, "Electroencephalographic changes in acute cerebral anoxia from cardiac or respiratory arrest," *Electroencephalography and Clinical Neurophysiology* 18 (1965): 575–86; J. F. Alderete, F. R. Jeri, E. P. Richardson Jr., S. Sament, R. S. Schwab, and R. R. Young, "Irreversible coma: a clinical electroencephalographic and neuropathological study," *Transactions of the American Neurological Association* 93 (1968): 16–20.

43. Alderete et al., "Irreversible coma."

44. Hockaday et al., "Electroencephalographic changes in acute cerebral anoxia."

45. Adams, interview with the author, January 25, 1997.

46. William Sweet, interview with the author, April 22, 1998. Indeed, Sweet talked about approaching the criteria to make kidneys available. Given this advocacy, the rejection of his views underscores the peripheral importance of this issue.

47. Beecher to G. M. Williams, Professor of Surgery at Johns Hopkins, December 19, 1969, Box 13, Folder 14, Beecher Papers.

48. Adams, interview with the author, January 25, 1997.

49. Sugar and Gerard, "Anoxia and brain potentials," *Journal of Neurophysiology* 1 (1938): 558–72.

50. J. F. Alderete, et al., "Irreversible coma," 20.

51. Robert Young, interview with the author, April 30, 1998.

6

Brain Death After Beecher and the Limits of Bioethics

"The concept of brain death remains incoherent...by abandoning the concept...we may be able to increase both the supply of transplantable organs and clarify our understanding of death."

—ROBERT TRUOG, *1997*

"The whole-brain formulation of death not only is coherent, but remains closest to our traditional concept of death."

—JAMES L. BERNAT, *1998*

"For "problems of wicked complexity...muddling through is not a second best process to be dropped once optimization techniques are developed...It is the best we can do.""

—BRADEN R. ALLENBY AND DANIEL SAREWITZ, *2012*

The predominant historical characterization of the Harvard Report as inattentive to the conceptual or ethical dimensions of its work, lacking empirical grounding, and motivated to harvest organs, does not hold. More than that, the history described in this book questions a central tenet of bioethics—that a vacuum of ethical expertise is at the root of medical dilemmas—evident throughout canonical histories of the field.[1]

The path taken by several decades of bioethical critique and debate over brain death only underscores skepticism over the supposedly unique need for or value of bioethics. Debate after Beecher cycled through a fairly narrow set of vying concepts to describe life, death, and consciousness, and didn't travel much beyond the concepts that Schwab, Beecher, and 1950s RAS researchers used except that the latter stayed closer to real bodies and how they worked. *Their* path, grounded in practice, reinforced the notion that medical dilemmas are driven by the more enduring challenges and questions raised by medical knowledge and its use: How well do we know what we think we know when we try to manage ourselves as biological things? What anxieties and uncertainties arise when doing so? How do the priority questions and aims that drive what knowledge we look for get selected? How are those constrained socially, and by the limits of the existing capabilities, tools, knowledge, and outcomes that we have? There are ethical aspects of these questions to be sure, as there are to everything. But while these are evidentiary, existential, psychological, technical, phenomenological, experiential, and sociological challenges, they are not essentially or primarily best approached or framed as ethical ones.

While in the United States and elsewhere new ethics review procedures and rules of thumb did become widespread in medical practice, these procedures—which included routine written consent, assigned proxy, and respect for autonomy—were arguably reflections of changing legal and judicial action across a range of similar rights, and shifts in social norms around authority and civil liberties. Further historical scholarship is needed to better understand how and whether these developments led or followed the establishment of a unique ethical expertise. Little in the way of empirical evidence, or methods to gather it, were developed or sought during this period to capture the impact or added value of the work of bioethics. More specifically, we know little about the connection between healthcare ethics consultation (HCEC) and medical effectiveness, patient benefit, or knowledge of ethics for that matter. A review of HCEC competencies by the American Society for Bioethics and Humanities concluded, for example, that "the Task Force did not locate evidence that HCEC actually improved ethics knowledge."[2]

The investment of energy and attention to medical ethics—in this case in what something like brain death *means* rather than what it *does*—was mirrored in a national political culture in the United States that was ambivalent about rationalizing healthcare. That ambivalence allowed for exponential growth in medical care investments without achieving commensurate improvements in health. Contradictory expectations about technologically intensive medicine—that it be more powerful but less intrusive, more sophisticated but not expert-driven, less costly but available without restrictions, mission-driven but lucrative and market driven—reflect marginalization of the question of what we want medicine to do. The wish that individual choice might manage that question, as well as take on the complexity and consequences of medicine's technologically driven history, was and remains insufficient. Individual choice, whether in the version of patient autonomy as a sufficient answer to difficult decisions, or as an idealized consumer somehow navigating complex healthcare management, proved unable to live up to expectations. The patient-autonomy version positioned ethics as an awkward and indirect language to use to clarify the ends and content of medicine. The consumerist version did its part to help drive the implosion of US healthcare as a cost-effective enterprise since the 1970s. The increasingly pressing question of how to square healthcare with values requires different tools that more directly and substantively take on the management and use of medical knowledge.

The potential for the new bioethics movement to be part of taking that on was diminished early. Veatch's shift—from looking for thick and precise sociological descriptions of differently situated roles that framed medical evidence, to thin conceptual descriptions of medical categories without grounding in observation and data—is emblematic of that lost potential. This was a consequential shift from curiosity about how medical knowledge is generated and used (and how it can and should be leveraged better), to a pretense for replacing it.

MEDICAL FACTS: THE CALCULUS OF SURVIVAL

The path taken by the Harvard criteria after the Report appeared included restatement of its essential features by government review bodies and neurologist expert groups. A 2002 global survey of brain death guidelines in seventy countries, reflecting a wide range of social, religious, and historical cultures, found that while variation occurred in many aspects of the use of brain death criteria—such as the use of confirmatory tests, the intervals and frequency of examination, and who validated these findings—the key elements of irreversible coma—that is, motor unresponsiveness and absence of brainstem reflexes—appeared standard.[3]

Those elements first took shape essentially as an extension of Schwab's work at Massachusetts General Hospital in terms of discerning physiological survival in the context of the loss of a functioning nervous system. William Sweet argued that the key question the criteria faced in remaining valid was the strength of the assumption that it reliably excluded those who would continue to survive.[4] Several studies focused on the adequacy of physical examination versus ancillary tests and on technology such as EEG and cerebral circulatory imaging techniques. Electroencephalographers studied technical aspects of obtaining EEG in terms of avoiding misleading artifact and learning about the stability of EEG findings over time.[5] The predictive power of a single versus sequential EEGs and the minimum time between serial measures were frequent topics of papers, with large studies conducted in 1969 and 1970 by the Ad Hoc Committee of the American Electroencephalographic Society on EEG Criteria for the Determination of Cerebral Death. Schwab was a member of this committee and a co-author of its publications. Schwab included the preliminary results from the first seven hundred of these cases in his memo to Beecher, further encouraging a focus on defining coma. Based on these cases, he also advised that "there are those who say...that simple clinical judgment would determine the presence of irreversible coma. I think that is probably true, but the additional weight of EEG makes it conclusively certain."[6] That study eventually reported 2,650 unique individuals with isoelectric tracings. Only three survived, all of whom were within groups that would be identified and excluded from the criteria—in this case with nervous system depressant overdose.[7] Other studies supported the predictive meaning of isolelectric EEG.[8]

That cautious confirmatory check, and the lingering uncertainty about the answer to Magoun's question, would eventually diminish with further experience with thousands of cases. This experience, however, was slow to evolve. Initially, disagreement about the necessity, reliability, or sensitivity of EEG and the predictive power of physical testing of brainstem function drove work in this area.[9] Several studies argued that cessation of brainstem function alone, as determined by clinical examination, was indicative of death and did not need to include examination of peripheral reflexes or EEG, yielding what has been referred to as the *Minnesota criteria*.[10] Other reports concluded the opposite and supported Schwab's experience in how to be "conclusively certain."[11] In this context, the National Institute of Neurological Diseases and Stroke sponsored a nine-center prospective study of brain death criteria. Entitled the "Collaborative Study of Cerebral Death," its findings were completed in 1974, but the results were not published widely until the appearance of a summary report in *JAMA* in 1977.[12] What are the minimal criteria that effectively predict nonsurvival in a short period of time? Do these include EEG? What aspects of the physical examination are necessary?

Of 503 patients who met the study entry criteria—that is, they were unresponsive (no purposive response to applied stimuli, commands, or pain) and apneic (no spontaneous respiration and no effort to override a respirator for more than fifteen minutes), 90 percent died within three months. Yet only nineteen met Harvard criteria, if that was to include two isoelectric EEG criteria obtained twenty-four hours apart. If one isoelectric EEG was required in addition to the two study criteria, those physical signs together described 189 patients, 187 of whom died within three months. The two who did not die suffered from drug overdose and would have been excluded if dilated pupils were added as criteria. Thus the results suggested that unresponsiveness, apnea, dilated pupils, absence of other treatable cause (drug overdose, hypothermia), and one isolelectric EEG were adequate criteria.

However, while finding that the addition of one or more of each of the brainstem mediated reflexes (specifically pupillary, corneal, oculoauditory, oculocephalic, oculovestibular, ciliospinal, snout, cough, and gag and swallowing reflexes) "does not improve the accuracy of the diagnosis of brain death," the study concluded that "semantically, the absence of brainstem function, as demonstrated by inactivity of these reflexes, should be included in the criteria of brain death."[13] The group thus recommended as adequate criteria apnea, unresponsivity, the absence of the aforementioned reflexes, and one isoelectric EEG for at least thirty minutes' duration at least six hours after onset coma and absent intoxication, hypothermia, or other clearly treatable illness (e.g., cardiovascular shock). In uncertain cases, absence of cerebral blood flow was recommended to definitively establish brain death. Several decades later, US standards would step away from recommending an EEG as a necessary feature.[14]

A 1970 survey found that 28 percent of physicians would not turn off a respirator of a brain dead individual.[15] While on the one hand this reflects a huge shift in practice (two years after the Committee the vast majority of respondents presumably *would* act on these criteria), a sizeable plurality undermined claims to a background of full physician consensus. By the time Peter McL. Black, a neurosurgeon at MGH at the time, reviewed the status of brain death in the *New England Journal of Medicine* almost ten years to the day of the publication of Beecher's Report, the procedures necessary for predicting nonsurvival were still on the table—in particular the relative roles of EEG, physical exams and, with increasing prominence, blood flow imaging. The Conference of the Royal Colleges and Faculties of the United Kingdom required unresponsivity, respirator dependence, and physical exam evidence of absent brainstem reflexes. The American Neurological Association (ANA) accepted most of the "Collaborative" study guidelines but eschewed blood flow tests and trimmed back the list of brainstem reflexes to adhere more closely to the evidence. Sweet's accompanying editorial to Black's review gave him another opportunity to (unsuccessfully) argue for the British approach, and extended his dialogue with Schwab and Adams. An examination of brainstem functioning through physical examination was sufficient. EEG criteria narrowed the field of potential organ donors too much. The existence of nests of cells with some electrical activity did not indicate consciousness, and anyway was functionally inconsequential if the brainstem was nonfunctioning.[16]

Accumulating data continued to support and refine the prognostic paradigm, however, in that direction. In 1995 the ANA reinforced the whole brain criteria of apnea, absence of brainstem reflexes, and absent motor response (in the face of known cause, ruling out intoxication, hypothermia, etc., or other reversible causes).[17] A review fifteen years later by a subcommittee of the Academy identified no published reports in that interval that these findings were ever reversed, further narrowing the need for confirmatory testing and clarifying and updating evidence on the timing and frequency of assessments.[18]

Challenges to prediction of "survival" as a way to define death took on two basic forms. One was to report cases that questioned how reliable those predictions were. So, one forty-nine-year-old man in Syracuse, NY who met the Harvard, Minnesota, and NIH Collaborative Study criteria persisted on life support for seventy-four days, a streak interrupted only by a purposeful decision to terminate care. A published review of this case, however, did not consider it to question brain death but rather to reinforce the careful use of the criteria.[19] A more extensive and consequential analysis of outlier survivors—those with apparent brain death who survived for more than one week—was published by Alan Shewmon in 1998. Shewmon searched over 12,200 published reports on brain death and found 175 such cases of extended survival, 161 excluding those reports that relied primarily on media sources. Of these, about 80 percent lost cardiac function within one month, but approximately thirty-two survived at least four weeks, fifteen at least two months, and seven at least six months, with the longest at fourteen years.[20] Eelco Wijdicks, who advanced the ANA efforts at standardization, responded that Shewmon's cases reflected poor application and highly questionable selection of cases. For example, he argued that only two of these fifty-six cases included a specific report of recommended testing for apnea, and half the cases were reported through news, case reports, and letters to the editor, some of which included details that undermined the likelihood that a rigorous brain death examination was performed.[21] What is interesting about Shewmon's data is the purpose to which it was primarily put. That purpose reflects the more pervasive kind of challenge made to the logic of brain death than its predictive specificity. The acceptable boundaries of that specificity, and the overall problem of building knowledge that is in part predictive, offer concrete starting points to talk about a range of purposes and practices that enter into death-defining, and into medical care more generally under the conditions of of death before dying. Shewmon's data and the NIH Collaborative results should rightly fuel discussion about how medicine knows things, the methods for discerning the movements of biology in the signals of the body, problems of medical knowledge in its precision, the relevance of prognosis and conflation of omission/commission as features of medical action, etc. The use of Shewmon's data instead reflected a more common sort of challenge to brain death. It was used to test a *concept* against which the validity of brain death was presumed to be more importantly judged: that loss of "biological integration" was the *sine qua non* of death.

Rather than focus on the ontology of medicine, bioethics instead focused on describing and debating the ontology of death. While academic medical centers tested criteria against outcomes, a new network of bioethics scholars, reports, and expert groups generated a self-referring debate and cottage industry of books and articles around a "conceptual turn." The conceptual turn captures the ways in which the validity of brain death was understood to rest on assessing the consistency between the criteria and conceptual, moralized, descriptions of death. Decades of such effort yielded neither universal consensus over a conceptual description, nor consensus over criteria considered fully consistent with any of them. This failure was considered evidence among some that the criteria themselves were unsupportable, rather than casting doubt over this unusual method of conceptual description itself as the way to vet medical facts, a habit that arguably had been shed in the nineteenth century.

THE CONCEPTUAL TURN

The work of the "conceptual turn" focused on asking whether the death of bodies or persons should be the key focus for defining death, and what if anything consequentially distinguished one from the other. Arguments both supporting and questioning brain death also regularly turned on whether it was preferable or possible to strip away the medical context of life support to reach the "real" nature of death.

Veatch perhaps most vigorously kicked off the conceptual turn in forums and papers, claiming that the definition of death relied on philosophically derived meanings and conceptual categories, not medical judgment or evidence. As mentioned, he elaborated perhaps most fully in his first major book that death had been characterized conceptually as four general types through history.[22] These types were: loss of a soul, loss of fluid flow, loss of integration of functioning, and loss of social interaction. Death was arguably many things depending on one's premises, and despite Veatch's increasing disappointment in the "whole" brain criteria and his support for a "higher" one, he advocated the possibility that persons could elect, while competent, the standard with which their death would be determined. Autonomous choice defined death.

The first Hastings Center study of brain death focused as well on the idea that the key task of the emerging bioethics expert was to clarify the conceptual underpinnings of a brain death definition.[23] Alexander M. Capron directed the President's Commission on Ethical Problems in Medicine and Biomedical and Behavioral Research, strongly shaping its conclusion about brain death as conceptually no different than heart-based definitions.[24] At about the same time, in 1972, he wrote an influential paper in the *University of Pennsylvania Law Review* with Leon Kass. With Kass, Capron was also a founding Fellow at Hastings and would serve on its board. In this paper, they feared an already-proliferating menu of conceptualizations of death and advanced one operative concept based on the "fact" that the brain death criteria were an extension of the traditional heart-based one.[25] That concept (or "fact"?) proved perhaps the most durable and influential, but a proliferation of conceptual branding rather than consensus characterized the following decades. At the first Hastings Center meeting on the topic of brain death—where participants were unable to arrive at a consensus on the underlying justificatory concept of death, but were firm nevertheless in asserting the publicly deliberated need for one—one attendee described the lack of consensus this way:

> [Some] held that a definition of death should answer the question: "When does it no longer make sense to think of a person— whether conceived as an experience, or an agent or a member of the moral community—as being in the world?" "We do not," it was argued, "want to confuse persons with things, including merely biologically alive things." Other participants objected, emphasizing a critical distinction between the "class of moral agents" and "human beings," and arguing that personhood is not the appropriate language on which to base a definition of death.[26]

The conversation remained essentially the same after the meeting, deepening the ruts of a well-traveled mind-body Cartesian divide. This mind/ body, person-centered/organism-centered division was often reduced to the highly inaccurate anatomical catch phrases or analogies of "higher" and "lower"—or, to include both, "whole" brain—standards. The "higher" camp tended to build upon an argument, typically elaborated early on by Green and Wikler, that loss of personal identity was the fundamental aspect of death, and as such constituted the ethical justification for brain death criteria. From their perspective, the "lower" brain death approach was, regrettably, what Capron and Kass said it was—an attempt to keep brain death conceptually equivalent to heart-lung death, an accusation that was also often directed at whole-brain advocates. Brain death, their argument went, emerged instead precisely to correct, not simply update, the limitations of that heart-based concept. In a series of thought experiments involving transplanted heads and considerations of who was who and what was what as a consequence, Green and Wikler, and many authors following this sort of hypothetical creativity, concluded that the heart-lung and "lower" views did not capture what we mean when we consider a person to be dead. That is, we look for the presence of personhood, of personal identity.[27] The definition of death, they argued, should reflect that. That argument also implicitly if not explicitly considered centuries of heart-based death pronouncing, what other critics saw the criteria as upending rather than reinforcing, were conceptually misguided.

The response to this personhood-matters position essentially went like this: Even if one conceded that personhood was central and was also reducible to awareness of identity, the loss of which could be convincingly located in either brainstem or neocortical damage, such loss was hard to measure reliably and was also not equivalent to *death*. Death didn't take place at the level of a person but of an organism. It needed to be described based on how an organism functions.[28] Early on in this debate, Lawrence Becker elaborated on what it meant. Death was not a failure of one capacity of the organism. The loss of consciousness was no more death than was loss of a limb. The relevant loss was when homeostatic processes were irreversibly lost. That, however, was not always a clear point with regard to time, biology, or criteria.[29]

In perhaps the most influential version of this organism-integrity approach, James Bernat, Charles Culver, and Bernard Gert argued similarly that death must be a statement about biological functioning, not a psychological concept. The latter was too imprecise to define. Death was the "permanent cessation of functioning of the organism as a whole." In the early 1970s Bernat, a neurologist, reached out to his Dartmouth colleagues when planning a grand rounds to consider this "new idea of brain death...as we weren't sure if they were really dead."[30] Gert was a moral philosopher interested in the relations between ideas about death and identity;[31] Culver was a psychiatrist and philosopher. The focus on integration, they argued, underlay the traditional understanding of death and implicitly required permanent, irreversible, and total loss of brain function.[32]

Improved ICU care replaced some of these integration functions of the brain. This was Shewmon's point. As bodies could be sustained for longer durations, and as irreversibly comatose bodies were discovered to still carry out some integrative physiological functions, such as temperature regulation, without the brain, did this then require, as physician Stuart Younger asked, "a more refined definition that emphasizes functions that cannot be replaced through technology[?]"[33] Karen Gervais reinvigorated "higher" death views in large part by rejecting all this emphasis on biological integration, since the spontaneity of vegetative biological functions was of interest only when someone was not conscious, aware, or retaining identity. Identity was therefore more essential to our notions of death. Heart-based and brain-based concepts of death were not continuous or linked through biological integrity, but instead were opposite concepts according to this reasoning. Brain death required a theory of personal identity, a position that was, Gervais argued, the implicit basis of the Ad Hoc report.[34]

So the debate continued. Through this ongoing cycling and recycling of arguments, the tiny brainstem and the Report became stages for any range of positions. Arguments for the primacy of the integrity of biological homeostasis through "lower" or "whole" brain integrity on the one hand, as well as for "higher" consciousness and personhood on the other, could be projected onto the brainstem and onto the Report.[35] Increasingly precise attempts to distinguish the concept of persons from personalities, and humans from their bodies or from "humanoids," continued following the same basic rules of the conceptual turn: looking for natural or medical experience to match up against a conceptual description of what was lost in death. Twenty years after Gervais' case for higher brain death and Bernat's case for whole brain death, John Lizza summarized those arguments and the iterations in favor of them that had been recurring since. Lizza argued that two basic foundations for understanding death had emerged from this debate: either death was defined as the end of personhood or identity (often posited as different things), or as the loss of biological integration. Lizza further made the claim that these two stances could be reconciled. The first was too hard to pin down in standard measures or in precise criteria—was personhood (or identity) lost with the loss of mechanisms for memory, awareness, or responsivity? Was it even possible to test any of those mechanisms precisely? The second definition (loss of biological integration), was no longer a clearly distinguishing feature, as some capacity for "integration" demonstrably did not require the brain.

Lizza argued that a lot of ink spilled over these two key distinctions reflected confusion between the body and brain's *functional* and *substantive* aspects. Understanding these aspects could reconcile the dueling emphases on either the loss of bodily integration or of conscious functioning to describe death in terms of death of the *person*, since the body provides the substantive potential for both corporeal and psychological functions. Preserving corporeal functioning for its own sake mistakes a "biological artifact" created by technology with the kind of integration that matters in maintaining the core substantive potential of "psychophysical integrity."[36] Gert et al.'s integration mattered, but only in order to describe a body; integration alone was not sufficient to describe a body that was human, as opposed to a "humanoid" artifact.

This sort of attempt at synthesis didn't seem to move things forward much, but rather contributed to the longevity with which the conceptual project continued to circle back on itself. These decades of the conceptual turn also did not seem to move beyond the discourse they were ostensibly out to replace and correct. Schwab's distinction in the charts at MGH between clinical and physiological death mirrors the kind of integrity Lizza talked about, although with more empirically defined boundaries and signals. The research on RAS explored in Chapter Four harvested and generated a wealth of concepts, metaphorical language, placeholders about consciousness and the integrative functions of the brain, but it did so in order to connect concept, experiment, and direct experience with bodies. Jonas and Beecher engaged around the challenges to respecting psychophysical integrity in the medical context in ways that are still instructive. The repetitiveness of the basic arguments of the conceptual turn were generally matched by their distance from actual consequence. How does a psychophysical integrity concept translate into solutions and actions? How would practice look different as a result, and fit with other demands of care?

The conceptual turn lent authority to the method of reasoning by analogy, which elevated the use of brain death's conceptual meaning as the basis for evaluating the criteria. In a back and forth of opinions in the *Hastings Center Report* over the 2008 US Council on Bioethics findings reinforcing the "whole brain" Harvard criteria, Shewmon underscored the fact of variation in the biological functions still remaining in so-called "brain-dead" brains—the assumption being that such variation meant inconsistency and thus incoherence of the brain death criteria. He made the further analogy that total brain failure patients who had some intact and "holistic" physiological capabilities were comparable to embryos, in that their survival depended on connection via a "'tube' with a 'maternal ICU.'"[37]

It will take more than quotation marks to analogize an embryo and an individual who meets brain death criteria, sustained by a respirator expanding the lungs and pharmocologic micromanagement. In the development of these criteria, and most medical criteria, the desired precision of a medical fact is not based on a purity of fit but on the good-enough fit given its aim, results, purposes, current knowledge, and so forth. The degree of completeness of explanation, replicability, and homogeneity expected from that fact need only surpass the threshold where any incompleteness or variations become problems to the degree that they undermine the purposes or instrumental effectiveness of the fact itself. It may be interesting, but not therefore necessarily relevant to argue that not all brain dead brains were alike in these other ways. The significance of that variation is not found by mapping concepts but by describing how these sorts of differences matter to the purposes they serve and so how these variations related to other outcomes or mechanisms that the criteria described. The habits of conceptual purity and analogy, at least in the literature on brain death, similarly conflated different sets of therapeutic, functional, and knowledge conditions, such as the anencephalic and the brain dead.[38] Disagreement over the management of the persistent vegetative state (PVS), identified in the early 1970s, made use of analogies in ways similar to debates over brain death.[39] "Higher" brain advocates often reasoned that since the loss of personal identity was really death, then PVS patients could be treated as dead. But concept here also ran ahead of ways of knowing about consciousness. Some recent research underscores the distance between neat claims to "higher" function or "identity" and actual bodies by suggesting that at least some PVS-diagnosed patients express consistent responses to verbal communication, and so perhaps process language.[40] It is not clear yet what these findings say about the capacity these individuals have for consciousness. Describing that capacity will be a substantial challenge. Deeply held ideas and values about awareness, identity, or consciousness will of course shape how efforts to fill in such descriptions will unfold and be used. Describing the still dark world of PVS consciousness will best come from interactions between the social and cultural sourcing of those intuitions, and the capabilities and limitations of tools to pose hypotheses and draw evidence from biological systems. The conceptual turn overreached, and should not be resorted to for answers to these challenges ahead. It confused the contribution of critical reasoning to describe the social constructions and conditions that factor in pragmatic solutions to nature's puzzles, with such reasoning actually solving those puzzles.

ESCAPE TO AUTONOMY

The development of Non–Heart Beating Donation (NHBD) illustrates this overreach. I am neither advocating nor criticizing this practice, but commenting on forms of its justification. Eventually, ICU physician and ethicist Robert Truog, Shewmon, and others, advocated a return to a heart-based criterion because of disputed conceptual foundations.[41] The impression that conceptual consensus was not at hand carried enough steam to prompt the second US President's Council on Bioethics review of brain death in 2008. In the face of an opposing minority report, the 2008 review still endorsed the whole brain death criteria, although it modified the concept of brain-driven integration and described it as the "work of the organism *as an organism*... what distinguishes every organism from non-living... that is, receptivity to stimuli to act upon the world to obtain selectively what it needs."[42] These last words were essentially those of Adams's clarification of the criteria four decades earlier.

Despite the whole-brain consensus holding in the Council's review, the growing use of brain death globally, and expert guidelines reinforcing the cumulative experience behind it, decades of conceptual vetting of biological concepts began to erode its use—especially because of interest in transplantation. After reviewing decades of (repeating) debates over whole-brain criteria and over justifications for either a biological integrative function or a core personhood function, Scott Henderson succinctly captured the impact of this erosion and the logic behind it: [Since] "brain dead patients are not dead (i.e., the criterion fails to correspond to the definition), then the procurement of their vital organs for transplantation is the direct cause of their deaths."[43] Brain dead people, in this view, are not considered dead because the criteria fail a *discursive* test. And so because the criteria failed a discursive test, adherents to this logic can simply claim "brain dead patients are not dead," and so therefore there should be new approaches to harvesting organs for transplantation. Advocacy for NHBD—that is, the use of organs from non–heart beating donor patients—accelerated in tandem with this kind of dispute over brain death. In NHBD, organs are removed from someone whose heart recently stopped, usually in a controlled fashion. Heart cessation is controlled by planned treatment withdrawal in critically ill patients. It is decided and made to happen at a certain point in time. NHBD was and remains controversial especially since its adoption and advocacy through the University of Pittsburgh "Pittsburgh protocol," described and advocated in the United States in particular by Robert Arnold and Younger.[44] Criticism of the Pittsburgh protocol and NHBD surrounded its intentions to explicitly use patients as means, and left standing a still unanswered set of conceptual questions it was supposed to resolve: When does the patient actually die? How long does the *heart* need to be stopped before someone dies? When is such cessation irreversible? The apparent solution to one conceptual quagmire, which justified NHBD in the first place, produced another. As Beecher also wondered in a 1970 letter to Harvard colleague and anthropologist Arthur Dyck, "I do not understand why death of the brain, of the person, of the personality, raises any more questions of 'profoundly theoretical and moral' issues than does death of the heart."[45]

Arnold and others found a solution to this potentially endless back-and-forth of conceptual hits and volleys in the idea of autonomy. Consent, by the patient or his/her family, resolved uncertainty over when to time irreversible of loss of cardiac function, or more practicably, how long to wait after the heart stopped to retrieve organs. Arnold summarized this position in the Institute of Medicine (IOM) report that established initial national guideline recommendations for NHBD in the United States in 1997: "[E]ven if the cessation could be reversed, it can be defined as irreversible because a decision has been made not to resuscitate. These patients have decided, or their families have decided, that they will forgo life-sustaining treatment."[46] So criticism of the conceptual failures of the Harvard Report, which was an effort to define the limits of death by authors *incidentally* concerned with and even wary of transplantation, justified an approach to defining death *primarily and overtly* intended to advance transplantation. With a logic reminiscent of precisely the kind of arbitrariness and self-serving utilitarian calculus Beecher was accused of wielding, the potentially difficult questions of irreversibility and heart-based death were superseded by the principle of consent. Failed expectations of conceptual consistency undermined brain death, but then selectively rescued a desired practice—gaining access to more organs for transplant—by drawing on another conceptual device, the autonomous person.

This was precisely the sort of appeal to autonomy that Beecher and his contemporaries worried about—that consent alone would be used to fast-track the physicians' ability to use patients for others' ends. As Beecher argued, "not any ends counted." Whether NHBD lives up to its ends, as Beecher challenged brain death to do, is an answerable question, and should be a very public one. It has not been. We have to wonder if that is in large part due to the new habit of outsourcing the hard choices over medicine's purposes to a process of conceptual vetting, or of deferring them to autonomous patients or their proxies to solve. Henderson acknowledged some of the questions NHBD posed, but pointed out a typical response:

No policy proposal is without its problems. Rather this rationale paves the way for the implementation of social policy with the aim of

accomplishing that for which the brain-death criterion was created, apart
from the vast majority of ethical problems with which it is associated.[47]

Yet brain death wasn't, at its origins, "created" for this "social policy" purpose of getting transplants. Its "ethical problems" were only problems as
such within self-validating subjective tests of conceptual categories and
analogies to make moral arguments. Henderson's position—that brain
death was crafted by the Committee primarily if not solely to advance
transplantation—involved quoting others' limited accounts, and citing
what was actually Curran's rejected Memorandum as if it were an early
draft of the report in order to establish an apparently key "smoking gun" of
interest in transplantation. Without attribution, he insisted that unnamed
transplant surgeons had pressured the Committee to revise a seventy-two-
hour criterion for repeat examination down to twenty-four hours. As is
clear from MGH records, the twenty-four-hour practice drove Schwab's
routine, and the Committee did not consider a seventy-two-hour mar-
gin. To assert historical precedent for NHBD, pre-brain death transplant
surgeons were characterized as essentially turning off life support, waiting briefly, and removing organs. This historical characterization was also
typical in the resurgent advocacy for controlled death practices in the
1990s. But this was hardly a norm, let alone an acceptable one. The risks
of that were widely identified among both legal experts and surgeons, as
described in Chapter Three.

A self-referring practice of concept-vetting, supported by thin and
inaccurate uses of history, helped drive the promulgation of NHBD and
questions over brain death. When more carefully engaged, what instead
emerges from that history is an alternative to the conceptual turn for
managing the unavoidable element of "arbitrariness" and value in medical
facts. Beecher valued the parsing of means and ends, in order to justify
the use of hybrid facts that were both objectively testable and contextually
instrumental. Beecher engaged in the processes of testing and evaluating
bodies that lay at the core of pragmatic medical knowledge-making. These
values and methods seem worth at least considering as alternatives to the
conceptual turn.

Indeed, my own emphasis on the contingent practice origins of brain death criteria and their validation suggests, even predicts, that the criteria and its use would change over time. The issue, though—and it affects an array of decisions about medical values and practices—is with what evidentiary and empirical tools and starting point of view do we use to make, or notice, those changes?

Beecher could be seen as choosing between Paul Ramsey's caution that our bodies set limitations on our choices and Joseph Fletcher's assertion of true freedom in our efforts to overcome those limitations. Bioethicist and moral theologian Gilbert Meilander framed the debate this way:

> It is not too much to say that two quite different visions of the person—Fletcher's and Ramsey's—have been at war with each other during the three decades or so that bioethics has been a burgeoning movement. But it is equally clear that one view has begun to predominate within the bioethics world and perhaps within our culture more generally.[48]

Meilander worried that the ascendant view was Fletcher's. Relying on choices by autonomous agents to define ethical actions simply came up short in helping to manage issues like PVS and brain dead patients. To describe an ethics of care in these situations required a return to beneficence, to physician judgment about the state and trajectory of the body, in order to "recapture the connection between our person and the natural trajectory of bodily life."[49] Fletcher, however, likely agreed with Meilander more than he realized. Fletcher recognized that the practice of medicine and the increasing application of complex technologies to advance health complicated any idea of a "natural trajectory of bodily life." Rather than shrink from this development into the equally arbitrary notions of "human nature" that Fletcher accused Ramsey and others of settling for, we need to live up to our ability to alter life's trajectory and, in doing so, to describe human nature in the most tangible, replicable, and transparent terms we can. This is what medicine does (or should do), and it requires more, not less, expert input as to the costs, benefits, and capabilities of medical knowledge and technologies. Relatedly, patient choices cannot be framed *simply* as a matter of autonomy. In this regard, Fletcher could have agreed with Meilander's concern that by placing autonomy at "the center of our understanding of personhood" and, moreover, "having used patient autonomy as a hammer to bludgeon into submission paternalistic physicians, we suddenly rediscover the responsibility of physicians to consider what is really best for the patient, to make judgments when care is futile."[50]

More was at stake than an argument over this or that concept. Anxiety about the heightened strangeness of medicine was real, relevant, and was fueled by the conditions of death before dying. The conceptual logic behind NHBD is itself a consequence of how care changed—it has only further positioned death and dying to be so interconnected and proximate as to be widely open to manipulation—turning on or off at will—for various ends. This is why Beecher sought limits that were anchored and credible within a fabric of medical evidence and purposes rather than in autonomy *per se*. And this is why brain death became such an urgent and early grist for the bioethical mill, which tried, in response, to diminish the degree to which increasingly consequential medical facts were unstable, value-laden, and a source of anxiety. In the context of death before dying, ethical reasoning was held out as a possibile antidote. Bernat wrote:

> If we regard death as a process, then either the process starts when the person is still living, which confuses the "process of death" with the process of dying, for we all regard someone who is dying as not yet dead, or the "process of death" starts when the person is no longer alive, which confuses death with the process of disintegration. Death should be viewed not as a process but as the event that separates the process of dying from the process of disintegration.[51]

As Younger also noted: "Now we have the ability to tease apart the various components of human life... we are forced to choose among various functions and levels of organization of life, declaring death, sometimes, when life of some sort remains."[52]

This expanded opportunity "to choose" acknowledges the same kind of "arbitrariness" that brought Beecher criticism. That arbitrariness reflects the unavoidable contingency of biological knowledge based on what we ask and what we do to biological systems, especially our own, and thus permits an opening for social constructedness, cultural context, and interest-bias in medical facts. But in a pragmatic view of medical knowledge, that aspect of medical facts reinforces how these facts are indeed facts to the degree they also work socially—that is, the degree to which they do not, as described at the outset of this study, remain "mere data" but instead predict, enable, and attain consistency with actions we prioritize and care about. The degree to which medical facts are social facts determines a large part of their value and use. Lived experience, and the watching and counting and measuring and listening to patients, has to add up to instrumentally changing what happens to them in ways that matter. Brain death evolved from that sort of process and may further change because of it. This was recognized in Beecher's and Fletcher's pragmatism: "Facts are what their results are."

The social utility and context, as well as the testability and replicability, of medical facts are important resources for living with our biological selves. They are lost, or become exaggerated, when cleaving off value from mere data. The prominence of the logic of having "autonomy" determine irreversibility, as opposed to actually measuring patterns in heart function and conductivity, as the IOM Report on NHBD also recommended, reflects that. Part of the factualness of the brain death criteria came from its ability to align the actions of practitioners across widely dispersed places and to align, as well, knowledge about how the brain worked. It also came from the degree to which the criteria predicted and described tangible outcomes that made sense within a thick set of other facts and practices about death in medical care contexts and how the body worked. Medically treating a neurologically empty body made that fabric of practice incoherent to a broad range of medical, legal, and public stakeholders. This was not the result of a philosophical position around the ontology or basic nature of personhood or of the body, but of the ontology of medicine in place. Concerns about and even potential replacement of the criteria will most usefully be understood, discussed, and safeguarded, on that terrain.

Beecher sought Ebert's support for an effort that purposefully differed from the emerging bioethics approach to the value implications of medical knowledge. Beecher acknowledged that brain death was still new and that time would tell if it garnered the traction and social acceptance he assumed it would, given the conditions it addressed. He wanted to gather a group that differed somewhat from the Hastings gatherings (i.e., heavier on sociology than philosophy, anthropology than ethics) and suggested figures such as Arthur Dyck, Renee Fox, and Stanley Reiser (and, of course, Fletcher and Adams) to think about and prepare for the ways that brain death would "surely entail some great changes in medical principle and medical practices. In an effort to gain greater insight as to what these changes will be," Beecher continued in his letter to Ebert, "I have gathered together a small group to explore informally the future possibilities."[53] To Fox, he lamented: "I am in a state of considerable uncertainty regarding Dan Callahan's group. That group seems to be on a tack where I can make no contribution...I still think we talk words when we should be talking about things—at least part of the time."[54]

As Eric Racine carefully described, a tension over the role of naturalism in bioethics has long been present in that field. Biological naturalism describes an approach in which biological and natural facts are the predicates and starting points for determining what is ethical. The moral "ought" follows from the natural "is." Inclusion of natural facts in ethics doesn't require, though, having to choose between a "strong naturalism" or an anti-naturalism, where ethical concepts are absolutely nonnatural—in other words, *ought* is not at all deducible from *is*. Instead, Racine described an often-implicit middle ground of "moderate pragmatic naturalism" or MPN, where *ought* makes sense in a context of what is. What Racine describes as MPN seems is conversant with Beecher's pragmatism and his referencing of Bronowski with respect to the role of science for framing values.

It is unclear though, in light of these frameworks, what ethics then adds. The conceptual turn was positioned off to the nonnaturalist side of MPN and attempted to crowbar medical facts outside of the context that made them factual. A 1989 survey by Younger found that clinicians declaring death and other healthcare providers working with comatose and vegetative patients had disparate notions of what brain death entailed, often understanding it as solely loss of consciousness, treating a patient as dead whom they felt was really dying, and using the concept inconsistently.[55] The survey, while taken to undermine the conceptual rigor of brain death, begged the question as to whether conceptual diversity tells us what we need to know about empirical inadequacy. Similarly, agreement on facts is possible without agreement on concepts. Research on RAS again is an example of how theoretical and conceptual diversity generated further working knowledge precisely because of reference along shared sets of findings and physical events. Brain death and most medical facts may be conditional, or conceptually untidy, but not in ways that ethical tools are able or best positioned fix.

A more sweeping indictment of the Western phenomenon of ethics as a field dislodged from the conditions of usable knowledge is found in Alasdair MacIntyre's *After Virtue*, first published in 1982. MacIntyre used an imaginary scientific catastrophe to analogize the predicament of modern ethics' relationship to perceived reality. Imagine, he wrote, that scientific institutions are discontinued and books and institutions are destroyed or outlawed, but then picked up again centuries later. People would learn and discuss "science" from fragments of books and repeat the surface instructions of experiments without knowledge of what they were used for or to whom they were speaking, and without context for the purposes for which these experiments made sense. People might recite and memorize the periodic tables or geometric theorems and attain a certain level of coherence in discussing these terms without realizing that they weren't doing science at all. They could debate meanings of neutrinos, mass, and so on without actually using or engaging with these concepts materially; philosophers would subsequently offer varying ideas as to what these competing views of neutrinos, mass, and so forth really consisted. These imaginary philosophers could even have metaphysical discussions over the role of realism or subjectivism in these matters. Moral argument would appear to hold knowledge about something when, substantially, it did not. The current language and analysis of morality is like this, MacIntyre argued: "the language of morality is in the same state of grave disorder as the language of natural science in the imaginary world which I described. What we possess...are the fragments of a conceptual scheme. We posses simulacra of morality."

MacIntyre captured what he saw as the failures of the Western project of ethics as it formed in roughly the seventeenth through nineteenth centuries, failures that lay in trying to be something that it is not. In that period, "morality" carved its own space as a cultural mode for describing credible action that was not based in theology, legality, or aesthetics, but was justified instead in rational analysis. To get there, though, the way in which definitions of "good" had previously attained efficacy and power—a social trajectory that started with description, knowledge, and understanding, and continued via the pursuit of practices and virtues—was lost. The new Rational argument, which accounted for ethics by way of reason, could not replace this prior process of determining "the good," which posited knowledge as internal to (and coeval with) practices. The notion of virtues provides a starting point for a more cogent psychological, cultural, and historical understanding of what is good; for a practical investigation of ethics and where it comes from; and for understanding what was lost through the Enlightenment revision of morality, which had another project in mind, namely the justification of autonomy. In short, the Enlightenment project was an attempt to achieve and create the socially and politically autonomous man using philosophy and moral forms of argument. These forms of argument, which I contend did not succeed on this small scale of medical value-making, MacIntyre concluded did not succeed on a grand historical scale either, as evidenced by "the gap between the *meaning* of moral expressions and the ways they are put to *use*." He continued:

> For the *meaning* is and remains such as would have been warranted only if at last one of the philosophical projects had been successful; but the use, the emotivist use, is precisely what one would expect if the philosophical projects had all failed.[56]

Neither I nor, I think, MacIntyre suggest that the autonomous mode is to be regretted or seen as suspect—just that it ought to be understood differently, as a historical not a rational accomplishment. It had a historical role and story that expanded voice and opportunity. If we are looking for a vibrant sense of the "good" in medicine, the starting point is to think seriously and expansively about cultivating practices that help us determine what that is. Repair of the separation of Beecher's "things" and practices from "goodness," and facts from values—unfortunate separations that the fragmented discourse of ethics reflects—can contribute to that.

It is interesting that early figures in bioethics often observed that medicine rescued a moribund moral philosophy from irrelevance—the irrelevance MacIntyre also consigned it to.[57] Rather than continuing to accept the application of moral philosophy to medicine as inevitable or even useful, we should be curious about why medicine at that time proved to be such an unusually fertile subject for it. Moore rejected the notion of the good as a definable category, arguing that it was only mistaken as such by way of the naturalistic fallacy; Kant attempted, instead, to describe how reason works, such that rules of morality work similarly in all of us. Both of these arguments seem to have to work too hard to rescue autonomy via methods of reasoning. Instead, the rescue of autonomy can and should be justified through what it does for us, or what we want it to do for practices that matter to us in ways that can be measured, listed, debated, tested, compared, and touched, like other things we make choices and set priorities about. In citing rationalism as a ground for agency, Aristotle spoke for a class of fourth-century BC Athenians, while Kant addressed emerging liberal individualism in the eighteenth century. Both of their claims and accounts for reason eventually returned to the formulation of knowing good within historically specific practices, goals, and actions. As MacIntyre described: "Any particular morality has as its core standards by which reasons for action are judged more or less adequate, conceptions of how qualities of character relate to qualities of actions, judgments, as to how rules are formulated, and so forth."[58]

Ethics and moral beliefs of right action are anthropological, social, historical entities; they are things people *have* rather than *prove*, and they emerge from relationships, roles, histories, and core psychological capacities. The focus by both critics and proponents of whole brain death on the ontology of death—that is, the description of the nature of what human death essentially *is*—diverted attention from the ontology and epistemology of medicine and the practices within which such a human nature is hammered out. What is the nature of this way of knowing, what kind of knowledge is it, what does it do, and how do we know how or whether it does this?

The degree to which the distracting power of meanings and morals may have also mattered on a larger scale bears repeating. The US healthcare system failed over this period to reach consensus on how to rationalize medicine, often turning to versions of individual autonomy as the solution. However easy to describe, the understanding of the patient as an autonomous decision maker (or consumer)—the main tangible impact bioethics had on medicine and medical research—has been far more complicated to achieve. It has, if anything, fueled the momentum of unconstrained ends. NHBD is a case in point. What begs our attention in that case, instead of rationalizations based on accounts or justifications of autonomy, is the way transplantation is valued and constructed as a practice (e.g., in terms of actual outcomes, impact on health, incentives of health providers, public attitudes, and so on). Beecher understood this.

So, after several decades of exhaustingly repetitive cycles of arguments over failures to unite conceptual definitions with a consistent criteria of death, it was brain death that was increasingly pointed to within this network of scholars as no longer tenable rather than the process of concept-criteria reasoning itself. The diagnosis of hypertension, or any number of other medical facts, would crumble under similar scrutiny. Defining when the force of blood against arterial walls constitutes a pathological deviation is conditional and has changed; the definition shifts with new evidence or from asking new questions, or wanting to achieve or being able to achieve new goals for health, and its criteria have been shown to be heavily observer-biased and subject to gendered, ethnic, and racial stratification. In this relatively simple task of defining of when blood pressure is "high," we see the interplay between normal and pathological categories, social and instrumental purposes and "mere data," as they yield facts internal to practices that work. We proceed to, and we need to, use this iterative, context- responsive, but hypothesis-driven approach to medical facts to manage our biological selves.

The original insight behind bioethics (that medical evidence ensnared values) focused less on trying to improve tools to act on the *relationship* between medical evidence and values than on *choosing* between them. A desired goal of autonomous patients and autonomous knowledge will always eventually bump up against constraints of the body. Those constraints give medical knowledge its structure, fueling ambivalence and anxiety about medicine but also providing the foundation of experience with bodily limitations that allow medicine to work—and make its workings sought-after. Gatekeepers of medical knowledge have been elitist, exploitive, unskilled, self-serving, and alienating, to be sure—all the more possible given the vulnerability that comes from illness, and more generally from ambivalent attitudes and deep anxieties about our biological selves and the complexity of medical knowledge. But the point here is not that use of medical knowledge can be elitist or poorly used—which it surely can be—but rather that its structure and rules are central to these issues, and must be engaged directly.

Beecher's and the Committee's work speak to the tight connection between ethical intuitions and the ways in which medical knowledge works—to the knowledge of good within the knowledge of practice. For an autonomous patient or concept of identity to be more than a figure of speech, or be justified by quoting Kant, the structure of medical knowledge itself needs broader and wider attention. Bioethics may in fact have slowed this down by driving both intellectual and actual capital into other, distracting questions, and by narrowing thinking about how to configure values in medicine.

In parallel with the development of bioethics were other, potentially more effective critical perspectives on medical work that emerged within the practice of medicine itself. Among these was an interest in understanding how clinicians went about knowing things. How did physicians use knowledge, test hypotheses, and deduce or induce a formulation about the nature of a medical problem and its preferred solution? Alvan Feinstein's *Clinical Judgment* in 1967 began to study how doctors drew conclusions and made inferences, and thus how they could improve outcomes, reduce errors, and promote health.[59] One can look back farther to the work of Ernest Amory Codman in the 1920s, whose "end results system" called for external monitoring of the objective performance and outcomes of surgeons. While resisted at the time, the system was nonetheless adopted and spread by some institutions and significantly influenced efforts to develop standardized evaluations of hospital performance that evolved eventually into the American College of Surgeons survey standards, the precursor to the Joint Commission for the Accreditation of Hospitals and Healthcare Organizations (JCAHO), which sets standards for most if not all US hospitals and many internationally.[60]

These sorts of developments reflect a potential but poorly explored, or as yet distinctly framed, theme and thread in the history of medicine: efforts to redesign medicine's effectiveness and accountability. Measuring "good" care (and also describing valued care) does not have to devolve into a straightjacket of data-driven inflexibility or scientism. Those risks are of course real, reflected for example in criticism of the uses and authority of "evidence-based medicine" (EBM) beginning in the latter twentieth century. But it is precisely in those debates over the nature and uses of evidence that people seeking care may be making deeper contact with medical knowledge, values, and expectations. The uses of EBM provides an underused opportunity to indeed better describe and work with the fact and value features of medical evidence, and to bridge clinical measuring and social sciences. EBM, treated as a form of reasoning, can be a point of entry for investigation of the relationship of medical to other ways of knowing, and of the social standards of medical evidence.[61]

Continuous quality improvement (QI) methods emerged to manage the twentieth-century transition from small manufacture to scale, and began to be borrowed from large industry and applied to healthcare in the United States in the 1980s. Indeed, a potentially important historical shift may have taken root in the late twentieth century, as medicine in the United States shifted in the direction of more broadly tying medical care delivery and design to accountable, public goals. QI was grounded in operations research and management science, disciplines that incorporated work in statistics, psychology, systems engineering, and iterative learning.[62] QI aimed to improve system performance in response to user-defined goals. Solutions come from harvesting local knowledge to literally diagram the skill, resource, process, or other drivers needed to meet explicit shared aims. This allows small-step, redesign and change initiatives tested in rapid turnaround pilot experiments—or "rapid improvement cycles"—to identify what works, relying on accessible and simple variation analysis tools that can empower a range of stakeholders to assess effectiveness and identify successful improvements. QI encourages inclusive, iterative, but empirically grounded knowledge-creation and learning about the work of healthcare. In 2012, the US Institute of Medicine explicitly supported that vision.[63]

A key entry point for the application of QI to healthcare came in the late 1980s with the National Demonstration Project on Quality Improvement in Health Care led by physician Donald Berwick, which in turn led to the creation in 1991 of the Institute for Healthcare Improvement (IHI).[64] IHI became a leading resource and facilitator of QI practices in the US healthcare system. QI was identified as a key tool to link cost efficiencies, clinical outcomes, and a good experience of care—what IHI called "the triple aim," a formulation that captures the key Institute of Medicine (IOM) goals of health system improvement with regard to safety, effectiveness, patient-centeredness, timeliness, efficiency, and equity.[65]

The triple aim and IOM goals seem quite similar to the pillars of principlism. Principlism described a formulation of the key features, or principles (autonomy, beneficence, nonmalfeasance, and justice) of ethical medicine generated early in the growth of bioethics in the *Belmont Report*. That 1979 report that laid the foundations for federal agency rules and criteria for ethics review of research on human subjects in the United States.[66] Principlism became, and arguably remains, a foundational reference point for work in bioethics and bioethics consultation. While quite similar, the elements of the triple aim are more clearly defined, actionable, and measurable. This is because they rest on more substantial expertise and knowledge-producing fields (operations research, statistics, psychology, systems engineering, adult learning, qualitative evaluation) going back to the early twentieth century.[67] QI may prove to be a better platform than bioethics itself to realize bioethics-inspired goals, to unpackage the individual and systemic sources that shape the uses of medical knowledge, and to sort out where the strengths of HCEC really lie.[68]

Similarly, "patient-centered care" has also been the subject of recent interest, and while the term captures a range of features it describes a potentially more complex and sophisticated project than "autonomy" as it includes re-evaluation of medical knowledge. Where successful, the features of patient-centered care have rested on evidence that they improve provable outcomes and are also cost-effective (the latter factor perhaps more influential in movement in this direction than moral philosophical arguments). The need for real innovation in the spread of far more participatory research or truly patient-inclusive treatment practices will find justification and traction to the degree that they perform as ways of knowing, rather than as ethical concepts. "Participation" will succeed where it contributes concretely to generating better knowledge and to informing and opening up the possibilities of doing so in instrumental ways that matter. How it indeed has that impact is a rapidly growing area of research and policy interest.[69] Strategies captured by patient-centered care, in order to be effective and grow, will not be essentially morally based but medical-epistemologically based. This is true as well for accelerated diversification in the last several decades over who is a medical practitioner. The focus of this history, and much of the history of medicine, on physicians, will increasingly look more broadly across types of health providers. Diversification of who can do what in terms of medical tasks is empowering and enhances access. But its growth has been fueled less by a driving ideology or moral commitment itself, than by experience and interest with how innovative re-packaging of medical knowledge can reach more people, more effectively, and with greater relevance to non-acute care goals such as to impact public health, function, prevention, and even social determinants of health.[70] Highlighting such goals requires political and social mobilization to be sure. But even advancing equal access to healthcare and to health for the specific purpose of providing "pragmatic solidarity" for social equity, begins with thoughtful and testable re-alignments of medical knowledge.[71]

While echoing goals that reach at least back to Codman, and relying on synergistic lines of work in multiple disciplines that reach back at least that far as well, the use of QI methods or patient-centered metrics is still new and its impact uncertain. Their appearance, however, demonstrates that we do not need to choose between describing medical knowledge as natural/factual or cultural/social, or get stuck in that divide. Embracing the dynamism of contexted and constructed, but also testable and often highly predictive, medical knowledge can keep us both on our toes, and well grounded in the world. Anthropologist Byron Good has pointed out that medicine can (and should) be a resource for acting on health and illness as complex facts, experiences, and aesthetics. Niche approaches to bioethics such as narrative or casuistical ethics share this insight. "Pragmatism," the knowledge of things in their consequences and application, came from the hands of Charles Peirce, William James, and John Dewey as a description of learning and cognition as much as a philosophy—and it turns our attention to practice. This helps explain why narrative, causuistical, and similar brands of bioethics have not taken on the complexity Good described in full—that is, their "way in" to that complexity is more descriptive than actionable, as yet unable to define, manage, or intervene in the very "structures" that they nonetheless acknowledge drive ethical commitments. As a consequence, these subfields of bioethics eventually fall back on MacIntyre's emotivist *use*. As Good noted several decades ago, "simply adding a bit of humanities to medical education or changing doctor's attitudes...is hardly what is at stake. We have a more important opportunity to help open up within medicine a region for vital research and practical activity."[72]

QI, participatory research, patient-centered and task-shifted care delivery that widen the idea of who provides care, and so forth, all reflect at least the potential for practical, grounded, ways into that complexity. Whether or not this proves to be the case, the thin line from Codman to Feinstein to Beecher to Berwick should be more deeply explored and filled in to better understand that potential.

MOVING BEYOND BIOETHICS

Criticism from within, such as Racine's, that bioethics relies too much on a too-narrow toolkit for analysis begs the more central question: Why?

Why, as Nikolas Rose put it, do we live with the "bioethical encirclement of biomedical and clinical practice"?[73] Rose described how "human beings in contemporary Western culture are increasingly coming to understand themselves in somatic terms: corporeality has become one of the most important sites for ethical judgments and techniques." A language of ethics and somatic self-identity have joined to arbitrate many aspects of modern life. As with "accountancy, legal regulation, audit and the like, [bioethics] has indeed become an essential part of the machinery for governing the bioeconomy, for facilitating the circuits of biological material required for the generation of biocapital, and for the government of all those practices in which life itself is the object, target, and stake." If "the forms of knowledge that are shaping our understandings of ourselves are themselves increasingly 'biological,'" it is not surprising then that ethics became more "somatic" and medicine more "ethicized."[74]

Sociologist John Evans, another keen observer of bioethics, has pointed out how the institutionalized spread and use of bioethics and HCEC rose in large part due to their ability to serve the interests of others (especially government research funders, courts, and health systems) by providing technocratic brokering rules for complex issues of agency and autonomy, especially with respect to human subjects research.[75] Doing so, as in Rose's scenario, may have then essentially submerged contentious questions and negotiations over performance, outcomes, priorities, and benefits by repackaging them as "ethical questions." Evans later argued that a more substantive claim for bioethical expertise and authority would rely on being convincingly able to use abstract knowledge to make recommendations that rest on general, logical principles and that credibly stand outside personal opinion or are at least accepted as such by the public.[76] How successful has that been?

Evans considers ongoing debates over the core methods of this evolving profession—such as recognizing limits to principlism and the possibility of situation ethics–based approaches—to reflect instability of the notion of a professional moral expert. As a corrective to this, he suggests greater use of social scientific methods. The relevant principles at stake in a particular issue, let's say defining death, may not be the same pillars of "principlist" bioethics that might apply to a different issue, but would vary depending on the context, consequences, and consensus around a given question. Survey and qualitative methods could be used to capture the relevant concepts held by the public, in this case about death, personhood, the role of the brain, and so on, as well as the principles they reflect. Principlism would be custom made for the issue at hand.

Evans seems to offer this "ground-up" strategy as a supplement to bioethical expertise rather than as a replacement for it. But his suggestion conflicts with what supposedly made bioethics distinct and legitimate in the first place: the use of abstract knowledge to make recommendations that rest on general, logical principles and that credibly stand outside personal opinion. To say, then, that this ethical system needs an empirical, not abstract, starting point in order to know principles gives away what it presumably "rests on" and how its conclusions derive authority. The use of abstract knowledge and the reliance on logical principles is implicitly then not enough, which is also seen in periodic calls for new directions such as "empirical ethics" among some sociologists and bioethicists.[77] The question—"why bioethics?"—persists.

Historian of medicine John V. Pickstone identifies how a series of distinct clusters of ethical, social, and scientific paradigms capture sweeping transitions in the history of medicine from 1700 to the end of the twentieth century. Taking his cue from the work of medical sociologist Norman Jewson in the way "he related knowledge production to patterns of professional work and power,"[78] Pickstone described what he calls four ideal socio-cognitive types—that is, distinct ways medical knowledge both made sense within and reinforced sets of social relations and values. The first type was the *savant*, which specifically reflected eighteenth-century European practice in which physicians were counselors to usually wealthy clients, and medicine circled around the individualized story of one's symptoms based on their life conditions, character, diet, and so on. For the savant type, the driving question was: "What have *I* got?" The *analytical* type captured early nineteenth-century Parisian medical innovation, wherein the relationship of physicians to the population and to bodies changed such that study of human tissue and pathology were referenced to explain the nature of disease. The driving question of this type was: "What is the composition of this specimen?" The appearance of experimental physiology and the possibility for more application of laboratory methods to care—due to institutionalized structures and expansion of hospitals' missions—was evident in the *experimental* type of the late nineteenth century. There, the driving question was: "How can we control this biological system?" Finally, the type that Pickstone (and Beecher) found themselves deep in the middle of was that of *techno-science*, accelerating into the twentieth century, in which increasingly capitalized medicine enabled more manipulative technological capability and offered rewards for using it as products from the laboratory became commodities. The organizing question of a techno-scientifically driven medicine, then, is: "What can we make?"[79] Along with this come the questions of what can we sell (or be reimbursed for by insurance)? These each reflect mutually reinforcing clusters of social roles, relationships, duties, and agreements as to how knowledge is attained and validated. These are thumbnail sketches, but powerful ones.

The rumblings of a potential though still evolving and controversial new type is perhaps discernible—one I characterize as *improvement*, driven by the question: "How can we find ways to have the best impact?" The joining of values of sustainability, efficiency, inclusion, and effectiveness as priorities for health systems globally are driving and being driven by a newly aligning Pickstonian cluster of concerns and practices, at the core of which is (and must be) an account of medical knowledge. In this improvement era, key concerns that have already emerged could include how to translate data-driven solutions for optimization to the level of individual patient care (as found in the use of and disputes over QI) or the capacity for converting complex biological knowledge into standardized work (as seen in the struggles over EBM). A potential "science of improvement" reflects the maturation of such concerns, and of methods that advance the "generation of practical learning that can be applied in real-life situations... generate local wisdom and generalizable or transferable knowledge... to form new synergies and release creativity alongside rigour... [and to provide] clear and explicit theories of how change happens."[80] Again, it is far from clear what direction these trends will take within a still contentious health policy environment in the United States. Their appearance, however, highlight alternative narratives and methods for moving medical knowledge in these directions.

The density of attention to ethics in medicine has no commensurate body of evidence to support its supposed value in protecting people or improving health. Its growth therefore needs other explanations. Here history is helpful. The turn to ethics fit well with the set of practices animating Pickstone's techno-science. It is uncertain how bioethic's technocratic functions in that context will realign within a Pickstonian improvement "socio-cognitive type," although calls for HCEC to serve the uses of QI as part of its scope and purpose suggest that this transition may have indeed begun or is at least possible.[81]

LIVING WITH THE WICKED COMPLEXITY OF BIOLOGICAL SELVES

Science offers a way to achieve scalable management of the contingency of natural events: "The history of science... is in a large part the history of the resources scattered along networks to accelerate the mobility, faithfulness, combination, and cohesion of traces that make action at a distance possible."[82] This presents both problems and opportunities, but will likely be a necessary tool for human civilization for quite some time. The predictive and manipulative capabilities and technical complexity of scientific activity can be used to silence other perspectives and advance some interests over others. But it can also anchor and allow transparent feedback and testable criticism to power. It offers the possibility for access to credible test beds for contesting and evolving assumptions about "what works." The key target at the outset of the bioethical critique—"medicalization"—is therefore a challenge to be managed, not simply named and wished away with dismay, or through ethical rules of thumb and deliberation. Rose again:

> Medicalisation has become a cliché of critical social analysis... But if medicine has been fully engaged in making us the kinds of people

we have become, this is not in itself grounds for critique. Critical evaluation of these heterogenous developments is essential. But we need more refined conceptual methods and criteria of judgment to assess the costs and benefits of our thoroughly medical form of life— and of those that offer themselves as alternatives.[83]

In their recent book *The Techno-Human Condition*, Braden R. Allenby and Danie Sarewitz described medicalization—indeed, a much broader and accelerated cultural biomedicalization—as "the techno-human condition." By this they meant the "achievement of new levels of direct control over the physical and cognitive performance of human beings, including the controlled biological evolution of performance standards, the direct intervention in brain function, and the gradual hybridization of human and machine intelligence."[84] If bioethics could not find common conceptual ground for explaining and navigating the definition of when death occurs, this new hybridization will prove much harder to take on.

Part of the failure of a moral evaluative response to a large challenge like this is that response operates mostly at the level of individual choice, and less often at a social level. Scaling up an individually coherent norm (e.g., "I have, or should be understood to have, autonomy to choose this") is hard to do because that norm behaves very differently at a more complex social level. Acting on techno-science primarily through *moral* or normative terms will fail: "We want to consider not what is technically correct or morally right…which only leads to [a] hotly contested but perhaps ultimately unproductive boxing arena as people defend their respective normative concerns—but what is, and is not, operationally feasible in this program of making humans better." It is not enough to just be mindful of these different levels at which technological practice acts; we must realize that these levels are incommensurable. Allenby and Sarewitz distinguished between Level I, II, and III impacts to capture how each level of impact from a given technology represents very different kinds of performance, metrics, management, and policy tasks. Level I involves meeting individual needs and choices (an automobile helps me get from here to there). That "ground-level" effect of a technology tends to lock in its use but then generates, at Level II, both unpredictable and far less readily manageable economic, cultural, and social practices and interests (malls and highway systems, energy supply choices, and delivery infrastructures); finally, at Level III, features of political economy emerge (mass-market consumer capitalism, environmental risks, class and gender mobility). Vaccines operate at these levels: to reduce infection, alter economic growth, and change long-term global demography and migration. Respirators do so as well: maintain cardiopulmonary function in an illness, enable nationally scaled harvesting and management of organs for transplantation, and finally, change expectations of citizenship and personhood.

Navigation around these choices and implications requires a range of tools and a sophisticated approach to science studies: systems economics, anthropology, participatory research, cost-benefit analysis, and so on. It requires careful attention to how we use facts and knowledge. Multilevel behavior—what Allenby and Sarewitz called "problems of wicked complexity"—stacks the deck against moral mapping getting very far, as such an approach cannot grasp this complexity and incommensurability. It cannot arbitrate the dilemmas posed by such incommensurability, as they argue: "a complex public health problem is nicely converted into a simplistic moral mapping by jamming a Level III system into a Level I simplicity."[85] Level I thinking seductively leads us to believe that moral language really tells us something useful. But instead, "[m]eaning, truth, values, therefore do not arise from first principles; they are…contingent and continually regenerated in a reflexive dialogue [with] external complex systems."[86]

The Techno-Human Condition and other works anticipate the kind of leaps and dislocating effects of manipulating the brain and cognition that also gave rise in the latter twentieth century to a new claimant as the pipeline for solutions to the complex challenges of techno-scientific culture: "neuroethics." While the term had been used before, this new field was essentially named by the Dana Foundation which jointly convened a conference with Stanford University and the University of California in 2002. That conference was promoted as marking a new discipline by *New York Times* columnist and Dana board chairman William Safire.[87]

The brain, and medicine in general, can be a seductive place for pondering meaning and for resurrecting faith in moral philosophy. Yet, experience with brain death cautions against squandering another generation of resources, including scholarly and policymaker attention. Likewise, we cannot afford to relay the message that the aspects of brain science most in need of public attention are ethical or are best managed through ethical analysis. It is better to address these new issues raised by neuroethics as problems of linking knowledge and aims. They are problems that call less for ethical analysis than broad literacy in how the relevant knowledge works or could work, assumptions behind methods of proof and framing questions (and which questions), and mapping the process and exchange of biological and social domains of knowing around neuro-scientific facts.[88] There are many examples of how much of what gets put under the new but already quite wide umbrella of work in "neuroethics," as with bioethics, is not scholarship or predominantly even ethics, but just good science or editorial writing—descriptive, informative efforts to capture relevant evidence, source implications, and give opinions.[89] The framing of that work as "ethics" is distracting, misleading, and creates distance—not participation, solutions, or rigor.

Medical knowledge needs to be put to better use as a resource for managing wicked complexity; far too often it is not. Instead of artful argument over a moral point of view, innovation and understanding of how medical knowledge works will be needed for real transformation and for the achievement of progressive values with which to navigate the continued intensification of biomedical culture, and the sometimes overwhelming combination of living lives of both agency, and embodiment. The ethical dimensions of all that are interesting but have not, and from experience so far likely will not, lead to the level of needed public engagement and intelligence around the uses of medicine and science.

Shigehisa Kuriyama beautifully explored what he called the "geography of medical understanding," spanning millennia and civilizations, as a way to capture efforts to compile knowledge of the working mechanisms of the body through touching and probing it in ways, whether in the East or the West, that were deeply contextualized and cultural and yet deeply empirical, tangible, physical, experiential, and verifiable. This is a pervasive, dynamic, and historically powerful form of knowledge, translating "the expressiveness of the body" into empirical knowledge that resonates with the most basic working beliefs of a society.[90]

Whatever values, interests, or abuses attach to the always imperfect but still quite instrumentally powerful fact-finding capabilities of medicine, the problems or prospects it offers should be engaged directly, rather than circumspectly through professionally derived rules governing discussion of morals and ethics. All dilemmas have moral dimensions. It is not clear, however, when they have or require moral solutions—that is, solutions primarily arrived at through moral analysis, reasoning, or related conceptual categories. The Committee reached their consensus through squaring medical descriptions of the body, with "RIGHTS." Looking back at what the Committee drew upon to define the complex fact of brain death complicates the predominant historical narrative of bioethical rescue. It directs curiosity and historical attention instead to the form and composition of medical knowledge, evidence, and practice itself, and how they contribute to and source values we want and need. These were and often still are the stated purposes of the medical humanities and social sciences, purposes overshadowed and diminished in the turn to ethics.

NOTES

1. Ruth R. Faden, Tom L. Beauchamp, *A History and Theory of Informed Consent* (New York: Oxford University Press, 1986); David J. Rothman, *Strangers at the Bedside: A History of How Law and Bioethics Transformed Medical Decisionmaking* (New York: Basic Books, 199); Albert Jonsen, *The Birth of Bioethics* (New York: Oxford University Press, 1998); Even critiques of bioethics also get the history of brain death very wrong, in ways that limit and distort the value and insights of these critiques. A recent example is a story of bioethics' continuity with eugenic and neoconservative market purposes, as argued by Tom Koch in his *Thieves of Virtue: When Bioethics Stole Medicine* (New York: Basic Bioethics, 2012). Koch's criticism of bioethics as over-focused on individual autonomy, with little to say about the larger population health needs and social and institutional dynamics that generate medical dilemmas to begin with, is an important and powerful critique. But to argue that bioethics had little to say about broader needs and

perspectives and yet was also the engine of efforts to advance statism, population engineering, and corporate interest, is difficult, just on its face, to accept as true all at the same time. One key element of Koch's historical argument that helps him make these connections regards brain death and the Harvard Committee. Koch uses the Report as a key example that supports his claim that bioethics furthered the dispensability of less-worthy humans for the benefit of the whole. As described in this book, more careful attention to both the evolution of the Committee's work and its bioethical critics, demonstrates that neither side fits that portrayal.

2. A. Tarzian, R. M. Arnold, K. A. Berkowitz, N. N. Dubler, D. Dudzinski, E. Fox, A. Frolic, J. J. Glover, K. Kipnis, A. M. Natali, W. A. Nelson, M. V. Rorty, P. M. Schyve, and J. D. Skeel, 2012, "Health care ethics consultation: an update on core competencies and merging standards from the American Society for Bioethics and Humanities," *American Journal of Bioethics* (2013).

3. Eelco F. M. Wijdiks, "Brain death worldwide-accepted fact but no global consensus in diagnostic criteria," *Neurology* 58 (2002): 20–25.

4. William Sweet and Charles Rich, "Development of criteria for the diagnosis of irreversible coma," *Transactions of the American Neurological Association* 96(1971): 314–17.

5. See for example J. K. Sims and Thomas W. Billinger, "Types of EKG Artifact Seen During EEG," manuscript copy, Grass Papers; E. O. Jorgenson, "Requirements for Recording the EEG at high sensitivity in suspected brain death," *Electroencephalography and Clinical Neurophysiology* 36 (1974): 65–69; E. O. Jorgenson, "EEG without detectable cortical activity and cranial nerve areflexia as parameters of brain death," *Electroencephalography and Clinical Neurophysiology* 36 (1974): 70–75.

6. Schwab to Beecher, May 14, 1968, Box 6, Folder 23, Beecher Papers.

7. Daniel Silverman et al., "Cerebral death and the electroencephalogram," *JAMA* 209, no. 10 (September 8, 1969): 1505–10, and "Irreversible coma associated with electrocerebral silence," *Neurology* 20, no. 6: 525–33.

8. C. D. Binnie et al., "Electroencephalographic prediction of fatal anoxic brain damage after resuscitation from cardiac arrest," *British Medical Journal* (October 31, 1970): 265–68; See also J. C. Mareska, J. R. Knott, and W. F. McCormick, "Electro-cerebral Silence and Pronunciation of Clinical Death," Manuscript, Grass Papers. This study reflected the experience of 120 patients at the University of Iowa Hospitals from January 1968 to June 1973; and P. F. Prior, *The EEG and Acute Cerebral Anoxia* (Amsterdam: Elsevier, 1973).

9. Donald P. Becker et al., "An evaluation of the definition of cerebral death," *Neurology* 20 (May 1970): 459–46; A. Mohandas and Shelly N. Chou, "Brain death: a clinical and pathological study," *Journal of Neurosurgery* 35 (August 1971): 211–18; Leslie P. Ivan, "Spinal reflexes in cerebral death," *Neurology* 23 (June 1973): 650–52.

10. Mohandas and Chou, "Brain death: a clinical and pathological study"; Georges Ouaknine et al., "Laboratory criteria of brain death," *Journal of Neurosurgery* 39 (October 1973): 429–33; and Korein, J. and Maccario M., "On the diagnosis of cerebral death: a prospective study of 55 patients to define irreversible coma," *Clinical Electroencephalography* 2: 178–99.

11. S. Lindgren, I. Petersen and N. Zwetnow, "Prediction of death in serious brain damage," *Acta Chirugica Scandinavica* 134 (1968): 405–16.
12. "A Report for the Collaborative Study of Cerebral Death: An Introduction," April, 1974. Manuscript Copy of the Chairman of the Editorial Board, Benjamin Boshes, courtesy of Roger R. Boshes, Harvard Medical School. The study summary appeared as "An appraisal of the criteria of cerebral death—a summary statement— a collaborative study," *JAMA* 237, no. 10 (March 7, 1977): 982–86.
13. "An appraisal of the criteria of cerebral death," 985.
14. Eelco F. M. Wijdicks, Panayiotis N. Varelas, Gary S. Gronseth, and David M. Greer, "Evidence-based guideline update: Determining brain death in adults—A Report of the Quality Standards Subcommittee of the American Academy of Neurology," *Neurology* 74 (2010): 1911–18.
15. Diana Crane, *The Sanctity of Social Life: Physician's Treatment of Critically Ill Patients* (New York: Russel Sage Foundation, 1975).
16. William Sweet, "Brain death," *New England Journal of Medicine* 299, no. 8 August 24, 1978): 410–11.
17. Eelco F. M. Wijdicks, "Determining brain death in adults," *Neurology* 45 (May 1995): 1003–11.
18. Wijdicks et al., "Evidence-based guideline update: Determining brain death in adults," ibid.
19. Joseph Parisi et al., "Brain death with prolonged somatic survival," 306, no. 1 (January 7, 1982): 14–16.
20. D. Alan Shewmon, "Chronic 'brain death'—Meta-analysis and conceptual consequences," *Neurology* 51 (1998): 1538–45.
21. Eelco F. M. Wijdicks, *Brain Death*, 2nd ed. (Oxford: Oxford University Press, 2011).
22. *Death, Dying and the Biological Revolution—Our Last Quest for Responsibility* (New Haven: Yale University Press, 1976).
23. Task Force on Death and Dying of the Institute of Society, Ethics and the Life Sciences, "Refinements in criteria for the determination of death: an appraisal," *JAMA* 221, no. 1 (July 3, 1972): 48–53.
24. President's Commission on Ethical Problems in Medicine and Biomedical and Behavioral Research, *Defining Death: A Report on the Medical, Legal, and Ethical Issues in the Definition of Death* (Washington DC: US Government Printing Office, 1981).
25. Alexander M. Capron and Leon R. Kass, "A statutory definition of the standards for determining human death," *University of Pennsylvania Law Review* 121 (1972): 87–118. See also Capron, "Determining death: Do we need a statute?", *Hastings Center Report* 1 (June 1971): 6–7.
26. Leonard Isaacs, "Death: Where is thy defining?", *Hastings Center Report* (February 1978): 5–8, 8.
27. Michael B. Green and Daniel Wikler, "Brain death and personal identity," *Philosophy and Public Affairs* 9, no. 2 (1980): 105–33.
28. George J. Agich and Royce P. Jones, "Personal identity and brain death: a critical response," *Philosophy and Public Affairs* 15, no. 3 (1986): 267–274.
29. Lawrence C. Becker, "Human being: the boundaries of the concept," *Philosophy and Public Affairs*, 334–359.

30. Personal communication, James Bernat, January 4, 2013.

31. Bernard Gert, "Personal identity of the body," *Dialogue* 10 (1971): 458–78.

32. Bernat, Culver, and Gert, "On the definition and criterion of death." See also James L. Bernat, Charles M. Culver, and Bernard Gert, "Defining death in theory and practice," *Hastings Center Report* (February 1982): 5–9; and Charles M. Culver and Bernard Gert, "The Definition and Criterion of Death," chapter 10 in *Philosophy in Medicine: Conceptual and Ethical Issues in Medicine and Psychiatry* (New York: Oxford University Press, 1982); James L. Bernat, "A defense of the whole-brain concept of death," *Hastings Center Report* (March–April 1998): 14–23.

33. Stuart Younger and Edward T. Bartlett, "Human death and high technology: the failure of the whole-brain formulations," *Annals of Internal Medicine* 99 (1983): 252–58, 253.

34. Karen Grandstrand Gervais, *Redefining Death* (New Haven: Yale University Press, 1986).

35. For example, David Lamb, *Death, Brain Death, and Ethics* (City, NY: SUNY Press, 1985); Agich and Jones, "Personal identity and brain death."

36. John P. Lizza, *Persons, Humanity, and the Definition of Death* (Baltimore: Johns Hopkins University Press, 2006).

37. Alan Shewmon, "And she's not only merely dead, she's really most sincerely dead," Letters, *The Hastings Center Report* 39, no. 5 (September–October, 2009): 6–7, 6.

38. Shewmon wrote poignantly about his experiences with anencephalic children he treated whose rudimentary brains could nonetheless perform purposeful tasks; this experience made him question whether consciousness actually only resided in the brain rather than being a more distributed property. He also questioned the ability to definitively isolate the neurological person from the functioning organism by seeing personhood in the organism's physiological vitality. Because of this, he abandoned his prior advocacy of first a "whole" and then a "higher" brain death standard. However, the kinds of combinations of injury and effects that entered Schwab's criteria were different. The analogy does not hold. D. Alan Shewmon, "Recovery from 'Brain Death': A neurologist's apologia," *Linacre Quarterly*, February 1997, 30–96. For a concise presentation of differing views on this, see a pair of *Sounding Board* columns: Robert D. Truog and John C. Fletcher, "Anencephalic newborns—can organs be transplanted before death?," *New England Journal of Medicine* 321, no. 6 (August 10, 1989): 388–90; Donald N. Medearis Jr. and Lewis B. Holmes, "On the use of anencephalic infants as organ donors," 391–93.

39. B. Jennett and F. Plum, "The persistent vegetative state: a syndrome in search of a name," *The Lancet*, April 1, 1972, 734–37; David DeGrazia, "Biology, consciousness, and the definition of death," *Philosophy and Public Policy* 18, no. 1–2 (Winter–Spring 1998): 18–22.

40. Martin M. Monti, Audrey Vanhaudenhuyse, Martin R. Coleman, Melanie Boly John D. Pickard, Luaba Tshibanda, Adrian M. Owen, Ph.D., and Steven Laureys, "Willful modulation of brain activity in disorders of consciousness," *New England Journal of Medicine* 362 (2010): 579–89.

41. Robert D. Truog, "Is it time to abandon brain death?" *Hastings Center Report* 27, no. 1 (1997): 29–37.

42. President's Council on Bioethics, *Controversies in the determination of death*, 60.

43. D. Scott Henderson, *Death and Donation: Rethinking Brain Death as a Means for Procuring Transplantable Organs* (Eugene, Oregon: Pickwick, 2011), 143.

44. Robert M. Arnold and Stuart J. Younger, "The dead donor rule: should we stretch it, bend it, or abandon it?," *Kennedy Institute of Ethics Journal* 3, no. 2 (1993): 263–78. For a cautionary if not opposing view at the time, see Joanne Lynn, "Are the patients who become organ donors under the Pittsburgh protocol for 'non-heart-beating donors' really dead," *Kennedy Institute of Ethics Journal* 3, no. 2 (1993): 167–78.

45. Beecher to Arthur Dyck, January 14, 1971, Box 13, Folder 16, Beecher Papers.

46. Institute of Medicine, *Non-heart beating organ transplantation: Medical and ethical issues in procurement* (Washington DC: National Academy Press, 1997), 86.

47. Henderson, *Death and Donation,* 168.

48. Gilbert Meilaender, "Terra es animata—on having a life," *Hastings Center Report* 23, no. 4, July–August 1993): 25–32, 29.

49. Ibid., 29.

50. Ibid., 29.

51. Bernat, Culver, and Gert, "On the definition and criterion of death," 389.

52. James L. Bernat, "Brain death—occurs only with destruction of the cerebral hemispheres and the brain stem," *Archives of Neurology* 49 (May 1992): 569–70; Stuart Younger, "Defining death—a superficial and fragile consensus," *Archives of Neurology* 49 (May 1992): 570–72.

53. Beecher to Ebert, December 22, 1969, Box 13, Folder 6, Beecher Papers.

54. Beecher to Renee Fox, May 17, 1971, Box 1, Folder 86, Beecher Papers.

55. Stuart Younger et al., "'Brain death' and organ retrieval—a cross-sectional survey of knowledge and concepts among health professionals," *JAMA* 261, no. 15 (April 21, 1989): 2205–10.

56. Alasdair MacIntyre, *After Virtue: A Study in Moral Theory*, 2nd ed. (Notre Dame: University of Notre Dame Press, 1984), 68.

57. S Toulmin, "How medicine saved the life of ethics," *Perspectives in Biology and Medicine*, 25 no. 4 (1982): 736–750.

58. MacIntyre, *After Virtue,* 268.

59. Alvan R Feinstein, *Clinical Judgment* (Baltimore: The Williams and Wilkins Co., 1967).

60. Christopher Crenner, "Organizational reform and professional dissent in the careers of Richard Cabot and Ernest Amory Codman, 1900–1920," *Journal of the History of Medicine and Allied Sciences* 56 (2001): 211–37.

61. Stefan Timmermans and Aaron Mauck, "The promises and pitfalls of evidence-based medicine," *Health Affairs* 24, no. 1 (2005): 18–28; Eric Mykhalovskiy and Lorna Weir, "The problem of evidence-based medicine: directions for social science," *Social Science and Medicine* 59 (2004):1059–1069; Dominique Behague, Charlotte Tawiah, Mikey Rosato, et al., "Evidence-based policy-making: The implications of globally-applicable research for context-specific problem-solving in developing countries," *Social Science and Medicine* 69 (2009): 1539–1546.

62. P. B. Batalden and F. Davidoff, "What is 'quality improvement' and how can it transform healthcare?," *Quality & Safety in Health Care* 16, no. 1 (2007): 2–3; D. Berwick, "The science of improvement," *JAMA* 299, no. 10 (March 12, 2008): 1182–84;

Rocco J Perla, Lloyd P Provost, Gareth J Parry, "Seven propositions of the science of improvement: Exploring foundations," *Quality Management in Health Care*, 22, no. 3 (July-September 2013): 170–186.

63. Institute of Medicine, *Best care at lower cost: The path to continuously learning health care in America* (Washington DC: National Academy Press, 2012).

64. www.ihi.org

65. Institute of Medicine, *Crossing the Quality Chasm: A New Health System for the 21st Century* (Washington DC: National Academy Press, 2001).

66. *Belmont Report: Ethical Principles and Guidelines for the Protection of Human Subjects of Research, Report of the National Commission for the Protection of Human Subjects of Biomedical and Behavioral Research.* (Washington DC: US Government Printing Office, 1978).

67. W. Edwards Deming, *The New Economics for Industry, Government, Education*, 2nd ed. (Cambridge, MA: Massachusetts Institute of Technology, 1994).

68. Gary S. Belkin, "Impact and accountability: Improvement as a competency challenges the purposes of bioethics," *American Journal of Bioethics* 13, no. 2 (2013): 14–16.

69. Joe V. Selby, Anne C. Beal, Lori Frank, et al., "The Patient-Centered Outcomes Research Institute (PCORI) National Priorities for Research and Initial Research Agenda," *JAMA* 307, no. 15 (April 18, 2012); Pamela N. Peterson, Susan M. Shetterly, Christina L. Clarke, et al., "Health literacy and outcomes among patients with heart failure," *JAMA* 305, no. 16 (2011): 1695–1701; Bridget M. Kuehn, "Patient-centered care model demands better physician-patient communication," *JAMA* 307, no. 5 (February 1, 2012): 441–42.

70. Prabhjot Singh and David Chokshi, "Community health workers—A local solution to a global problem," *New England Journal of Medicine*, 36 no. 10 (September 5, 2013): 894–896.

71. Paul Farmer, *Pathologies of Power-Health, Human Rights, and the New War on the Poor* (Berkeley: University of California Press, 2005).

72. Byron J. Good, *Medicine, Rationality, and Experience.* (Cambridge: Cambridge University Press, 1994), 181.

73. Nikolas Rose, *The Politics of Life Itself* (Princeton: Princeton University Press, 2010), 30.

74. Rose, ibid., 254, 256, 257. Rose's scholarship has for decades looked to describe the investment over the last several centuries in an understanding and experience of personhood, identity, agency, and citizenship through psychological and, more recently, neurological terms, and the implications for configuring power and authority in society as a result of that. Such terms have facilitated both empowerment and objectification in a broad array of contexts. See Nikolas Rose, *Inventing Our Selves: Psychology, Power and Personhood* (New York: Cambridge University Press, 1996); Nikolas Rose and Joelle M. Abi-Rached, *Neuro—The New Brain Sciences and the Management of the Mind* (Princeton: Princeton University Press, 2013). But in this research, Rose still sees an inevitable working through of social strategies of defining the self by way of these sciences, and also looks at ways of

describing and knowing our nature such that "neuroscience should become a genuinely human science." Rose and Abi-Rached, *Neuro*, 234.

75. John H. Evans, *Playing God: Human Genetic Engineering and the Rationalization of Public Bioethical Debate* (Chicago: University of Chicago Press, 2002).

76. John H. Evans, *The History and Future of Bioethics: A Sociological View* (New York: Oxford University Press, 2012).

77. B. Molewijk and L. Frith, "Empirical ethics. Who is the Don Quixote?," *Bioethics* 23, no. 4 (2009): 2–4.

78. John Pickstone, "From history of medicine to a general history of working knowledges," *International Journal of Epidemiology* 38 (2009): 646–49, 646; Norman Jewson, "The disappearance of the sick-man from medical cosmology, 1770–1870," *Sociology* 10 (1976): 225–44.

79. John V. Pickstone, "Ways of knowing: towards a historical sociology of science, technology and medicine," *British Journal for the History of Science* 26 (1993): 433–58; John Pickstone, *Ways of Knowing: A New History of Science, Technology, and Medicine* (Chicago: University of Chicago Press, 2001).

80. Martin Marshall, Peter Pronovost, and Mary Dixon-Woods, "Promotion of improvement as a science," *Lancet* 381 (2013): 419–21.

81. Anita J. Tarzian and the ASBH Core Competencies Update Task Force, "Health care ethics consultation: an update on core competencies and merging standards from the American Society for Bioethics and Humanities," *American Journal of Bioethics* 13, no. 2 (2013): 3–13.

82. Latour, *Science in Action: How to Follow Scientists and Engineers Through Society* (Milton Keynes, Bucks: Open University Press, 1987), 287.

83. Nikolas Rose, "Beyond medicalisation," *Lancet*, 369 (2007): 700–701.

84. Braden R. Allenby and Daniel Sarewitz, *The Techno-Human Condition* (Cambridge, MA: MIT Press, 2011).

85. Ibid., 64, 123.

86. Ibid., 186.

87. Conference Proceedings, *Neuroethics: Mapping the field, May 13–14, 2002* (Chicago: University of Chicago Press, 2004). An amazon.com book search of "neuroethics" as a search term in February 18, 2013 yielded sixty-four books—none published prior to the Dana Conference Proceedings.

88. Christian von Scheve, "Sociology of neuroscience or neurosociology?", in eds. Martyn Pickersgill and Ira Van Keulen. *Sociological Reflections on the Neurosciences* (Bingley, UK: Emerald Group Publishing, 2012), 255–278.

89. One of many good examples of accessible writing in this regard branded is Walter Glannon, *Bioethics and the Brain*, (New York: Oxford University Press, 2007).

90. Shigehisa Kuriyama, *The Expressiveness of the Body and the Divergence of Greek and Chinese Medicine* (New York: Zone Books, 1999).